DATE: _____ S M T W T F S

MUSCLE GROUP: _____ START TIME: _____

D1682843

STRENGTH TRAINING   HOW I FEEL: 😊 🙂 😐 😒 😣   WATER: oz oz oz oz oz oz oz oz oz oz

- [ ] UPPER BODY
- [ ] LOWER BODY
- [ ] ABS

EXERCISE	SET	1	2	3	4	5	6
	REPS						
	WEIGHT						
	REPS						
	WEIGHT						
	REPS						
	WEIGHT						
	REPS						
	WEIGHT						
	REPS						
	WEIGHT						
	REPS						
	WEIGHT						
	REPS						
	WEIGHT						
	REPS						
	WEIGHT						
	REPS						
	WEIGHT						
	REPS						
	WEIGHT						

CARDIO	TIME	DISTANCE	HEART RATE	CALS BURNED

MEASUREMENTS

NECK	
R BICEP	
L BICEP	
CHEST	
WAIST	
HIPS	
R THIGH	
L THIGH	
CALF	

NOTES/NUTUITION

DATE: _____ ☐S ☐M ☐T ☐W ☐T ☐F ☐S   WEIGHT: _____

MUSCLE GROUP: _____ START TIME: _____ FINISH TIME: _____

STRENGTH TRAINING   HOW I FEEL: 😀 😊 😐 😖 😠   WATER: 8oz. 8oz. 8oz. 8oz. 8oz. 8oz. 8oz. 8oz. 8oz.

☐ UPPER BODY   ☐ LOWER BODY   ☐ ABS

EXERCISE	SET	1	2	3	4	5	6
	REPS						
	WEIGHT						
	REPS						
	WEIGHT						
	REPS						
	WEIGHT						
	REPS						
	WEIGHT						
	REPS						
	WEIGHT						
	REPS						
	WEIGHT						
	REPS						
	WEIGHT						
	REPS						
	WEIGHT						
	REPS						
	WEIGHT						
	REPS						
	WEIGHT						

CARDIO   TIME   DISTANCE   HEART RATE   CALS BURNED

MEASUREMENTS

NECK	
R BICEP	
L BICEP	
CHEST	
WAIST	
HIPS	
R THIGH	
L THIGH	
CALF	

NOTES/NUTUITION

DATE: _____ S M T W T F S   WEIGHT: _____

MUSCLE GROUP: _____ START TIME: _____ FINISH TIME: _____

STRENGTH TRAINING   HOW I FEEL: 😊 🙂 😐 😠 😢   WATER: 8 oz. 8 oz. 8 oz. 8 oz. 8 oz. 8 oz. 8 oz. 8 oz.

- [ ] UPPER BODY
- [ ] LOWER BODY
- [ ] ABS

EXERCISE	SET	1	2	3	4	5	6
	REPS						
	WEIGHT						
	REPS						
	WEIGHT						
	REPS						
	WEIGHT						
	REPS						
	WEIGHT						
	REPS						
	WEIGHT						
	REPS						
	WEIGHT						
	REPS						
	WEIGHT						
	REPS						
	WEIGHT						
	REPS						
	WEIGHT						
	REPS						
	WEIGHT						

CARDIO	TIME	DISTANCE	HEART RATE	CALS BURNED

MEASUREMENTS

NECK	
R BICEP	
L BICEP	
CHEST	
WAIST	
HIPS	
R THIGH	
L THIGH	
CALF	

NOTES/NUTUITION

DATE: _____ S M T W T F S WEIGHT: _____

MUSCLE GROUP: _____ START TIME: _____ FINISH TIME: _____

STRENGTH TRAINING   HOW I FEEL: 😀 😊 😐 😣 😕   WATER: 8oz. 8oz. 8oz. 8oz. 8oz. 8oz. 8oz. 8oz.

☐ UPPER BODY   ☐ LOWER BODY   ☐ ABS

EXERCISE	SET	1	2	3	4	5	6
	REPS						
	WEIGHT						
	REPS						
	WEIGHT						
	REPS						
	WEIGHT						
	REPS						
	WEIGHT						
	REPS						
	WEIGHT						
	REPS						
	WEIGHT						
	REPS						
	WEIGHT						
	REPS						
	WEIGHT						
	REPS						
	WEIGHT						
	REPS						
	WEIGHT						

CARDIO   TIME   DISTANCE   HEART RATE   CALS BURNED

MEASUREMENTS

NECK	
R BICEP	
L BICEP	
CHEST	
WAIST	
HIPS	
R THIGH	
L THIGH	
CALF	

NOTES/NUTUITION

DATE: _____ S M T W T F S WEIGHT: _____

MUSCLE GROUP: _____ START TIME: _____ FINISH TIME: _____

STRENGTH TRAINING   HOW I FEEL: 😀 😉 😐 😠 😫   WATER: 8oz 8oz 8oz 8oz 8oz 8oz 8oz 8oz

- [ ] UPPER BODY
- [ ] LOWER BODY
- [ ] ABS

EXERCISE	SET	1	2	3	4	5	6
	REPS						
	WEIGHT						
	REPS						
	WEIGHT						
	REPS						
	WEIGHT						
	REPS						
	WEIGHT						
	REPS						
	WEIGHT						
	REPS						
	WEIGHT						
	REPS						
	WEIGHT						
	REPS						
	WEIGHT						
	REPS						
	WEIGHT						
	REPS						
	WEIGHT						

CARDIO	TIME	DISTANCE	HEART RATE	CALS BURNED

MEASUREMENTS

NECK	
R BICEP	
L BICEP	
CHEST	
WAIST	
HIPS	
R THIGH	
L THIGH	
CALF	

NOTES/NUTUITION

DATE: _____ S M T W T F S WEIGHT: _____

MUSCLE GROUP: _____ START TIME: _____ FINISH TIME: _____

STRENGTH TRAINING HOW I FEEL: 😊 😌 😐 😣 😠 WATER: 8 oz. 8 oz. 8 oz. 8 oz. 8 oz. 8 oz. 8 oz. 8 oz. 8 oz.

☐ UPPER BODY   ☐ LOWER BODY   ☐ ABS

EXERCISE	SET	1	2	3	4	5	6
	REPS						
	WEIGHT						
	REPS						
	WEIGHT						
	REPS						
	WEIGHT						
	REPS						
	WEIGHT						
	REPS						
	WEIGHT						
	REPS						
	WEIGHT						
	REPS						
	WEIGHT						
	REPS						
	WEIGHT						
	REPS						
	WEIGHT						
	REPS						
	WEIGHT						

CARDIO	TIME	DISTANCE	HEART RATE	CALS BURNED

MEASUREMENTS

NECK	
R BICEP	
L BICEP	
CHEST	
WAIST	
HIPS	
R THIGH	
L THIGH	
CALF	

NOTES/NUTUITION

DATE: _____ ☐☐☐☐☐☐ WEIGHT: _____
                              S M T W T F S

MUSCLE GROUP: _____ START TIME: _____ FINISH TIME: _____

STRENGTH TRAINING   HOW I FEEL: 😀 😊 😐 😒 😣   WATER: 8oz. 8oz. 8oz. 8oz. 8oz. 8oz. 8oz. 8oz.

☐ UPPER BODY   ☐ LOWER BODY   ☐ ABS

EXERCISE	SET	1	2	3	4	5	6
	REPS						
	WEIGHT						
	REPS						
	WEIGHT						
	REPS						
	WEIGHT						
	REPS						
	WEIGHT						
	REPS						
	WEIGHT						
	REPS						
	WEIGHT						
	REPS						
	WEIGHT						
	REPS						
	WEIGHT						
	REPS						
	WEIGHT						
	REPS						
	WEIGHT						

CARDIO	TIME	DISTANCE	HEART RATE	CALS BURNED

MEASUREMENTS

NECK	
R BICEP	
L BICEP	
CHEST	
WAIST	
HIPS	
R THIGH	
L THIGH	
CALF	

NOTES/NUTUITION

DATE: _____ ☐S ☐M ☐T ☐W ☐T ☐F ☐S   WEIGHT: _____

MUSCLE GROUP: _____ START TIME: _____ FINISH TIME: _____

STRENGTH TRAINING   HOW I FEEL: 😀 🙂 😐 😖 😫   WATER: ☐8oz ☐8oz ☐8oz ☐8oz ☐8oz ☐8oz ☐8oz ☐8oz

☐ UPPER BODY   ☐ LOWER BODY   ☐ ABS

EXERCISE	SET	1	2	3	4	5	6
	REPS						
	WEIGHT						
	REPS						
	WEIGHT						
	REPS						
	WEIGHT						
	REPS						
	WEIGHT						
	REPS						
	WEIGHT						
	REPS						
	WEIGHT						
	REPS						
	WEIGHT						
	REPS						
	WEIGHT						
	REPS						
	WEIGHT						
	REPS						
	WEIGHT						

CARDIO	TIME	DISTANCE	HEART RATE	CALS BURNED

MEASUREMENTS

NECK	
R BICEP	
L BICEP	
CHEST	
WAIST	
HIPS	
R THIGH	
L THIGH	
CALF	

NOTES/NUTUITION

DATE: _____ □ □ □ □ □ □ □   WEIGHT: _____
                       S M T W T F S

MUSCLE GROUP: _____ START TIME: _____ FINISH TIME: _____

STRENGTH TRAINING   HOW I FEEL: 😊 😌 😐 😖 😠   WATER: 8oz. 8oz. 8oz. 8oz. 8oz. 8oz. 8oz. 8oz.

□ UPPER BODY   □ LOWER BODY   □ ABS

EXERCISE	SET	1	2	3	4	5	6
	REPS						
	WEIGHT						
	REPS						
	WEIGHT						
	REPS						
	WEIGHT						
	REPS						
	WEIGHT						
	REPS						
	WEIGHT						
	REPS						
	WEIGHT						
	REPS						
	WEIGHT						
	REPS						
	WEIGHT						
	REPS						
	WEIGHT						
	REPS						
	WEIGHT						

CARDIO	TIME	DISTANCE	HEART RATE	CALS BURNED

MEASUREMENTS	
NECK	
R BICEP	
L BICEP	
CHEST	
WAIST	
HIPS	
R THIGH	
L THIGH	
CALF	

NOTES/NUTUITION

DATE: _____ S M T W T F S   WEIGHT: _____

MUSCLE GROUP: _____ START TIME: _____ FINISH TIME: _____

STRENGTH TRAINING   HOW I FEEL: 😀 😊 😐 😣 😠   WATER: 8 oz. 8 oz. 8 oz. 8 oz. 8 oz. 8 oz. 8 oz. 8 oz.

- [ ] UPPER BODY
- [ ] LOWER BODY
- [ ] ABS

EXERCISE	SET	1	2	3	4	5	6
	REPS						
	WEIGHT						
	REPS						
	WEIGHT						
	REPS						
	WEIGHT						
	REPS						
	WEIGHT						
	REPS						
	WEIGHT						
	REPS						
	WEIGHT						
	REPS						
	WEIGHT						
	REPS						
	WEIGHT						
	REPS						
	WEIGHT						
	REPS						
	WEIGHT						

CARDIO	TIME	DISTANCE	HEART RATE	CALS BURNED

MEASUREMENTS

NECK	
R BICEP	
L BICEP	
CHEST	
WAIST	
HIPS	
R THIGH	
L THIGH	
CALF	

NOTES/NUTUITION

DATE: _____ ☐S ☐M ☐T ☐W ☐T ☐F ☐S   WEIGHT: _____

MUSCLE GROUP: _____ START TIME: _____ FINISH TIME: _____

STRENGTH TRAINING   HOW I FEEL: 😊 😌 😐 😒 😠   WATER: 8oz 8oz 8oz 8oz 8oz 8oz 8oz 8oz

☐ UPPER BODY   ☐ LOWER BODY   ☐ ABS

EXERCISE	SET	1	2	3	4	5	6
	REPS						
	WEIGHT						
	REPS						
	WEIGHT						
	REPS						
	WEIGHT						
	REPS						
	WEIGHT						
	REPS						
	WEIGHT						
	REPS						
	WEIGHT						
	REPS						
	WEIGHT						
	REPS						
	WEIGHT						
	REPS						
	WEIGHT						
	REPS						
	WEIGHT						

CARDIO	TIME	DISTANCE	HEART RATE	CALS BURNED

MEASUREMENTS

NECK	
R BICEP	
L BICEP	
CHEST	
WAIST	
HIPS	
R THIGH	
L THIGH	
CALF	

NOTES/NUTUITION

DATE: _____   S M T W T F S   WEIGHT: _____

MUSCLE GROUP: _____ START TIME: _____ FINISH TIME: _____

STRENGTH TRAINING   HOW I FEEL: 😀 😊 😐 😕 😣   WATER: 8 oz. 8 oz. 8 oz. 8 oz. 8 oz. 8 oz. 8 oz. 8 oz.

☐ UPPER BODY   ☐ LOWER BODY   ☐ ABS

EXERCISE	SET	1	2	3	4	5	6
	REPS						
	WEIGHT						
	REPS						
	WEIGHT						
	REPS						
	WEIGHT						
	REPS						
	WEIGHT						
	REPS						
	WEIGHT						
	REPS						
	WEIGHT						
	REPS						
	WEIGHT						
	REPS						
	WEIGHT						
	REPS						
	WEIGHT						
	REPS						
	WEIGHT						

CARDIO	TIME	DISTANCE	HEART RATE	CALS BURNED

MEASUREMENTS

NECK	
R BICEP	
L BICEP	
CHEST	
WAIST	
HIPS	
R THIGH	
L THIGH	
CALF	

NOTES/NUTUITION

DATE: _____ S M T W T F S   WEIGHT: _____

MUSCLE GROUP: _____ START TIME: _____ FINISH TIME: _____

STRENGTH TRAINING HOW I FEEL: 😊 😃 😐 😖 😠   WATER: 8 oz. 8 oz. 8 oz. 8 oz. 8 oz. 8 oz. 8 oz. 8 oz.

☐ UPPER BODY ☐ LOWER BODY ☐ ABS

EXERCISE	SET	1	2	3	4	5	6
	REPS						
	WEIGHT						
	REPS						
	WEIGHT						
	REPS						
	WEIGHT						
	REPS						
	WEIGHT						
	REPS						
	WEIGHT						
	REPS						
	WEIGHT						
	REPS						
	WEIGHT						
	REPS						
	WEIGHT						
	REPS						
	WEIGHT						
	REPS						
	WEIGHT						

CARDIO   TIME   DISTANCE   HEART RATE   CALS BURNED

MEASUREMENTS

NECK	
R BICEP	
L BICEP	
CHEST	
WAIST	
HIPS	
R THIGH	
L THIGH	
CALF	

NOTES/NUTUITION

DATE: _____ ☐ ☐ ☐ ☐ ☐ ☐ WEIGHT: _____
　　　　　　　　　　　　　　　　S M T W T F S

MUSCLE GROUP: _____ START TIME: _____ FINISH TIME: _____

STRENGTH TRAINING　　HOW I FEEL: 😊 😀 😐 😣 😫　　WATER: 8oz 8oz 8oz 8oz 8oz 8oz 8oz 8oz

☐ UPPER BODY　　　　☐ LOWER BODY　　　　☐ ABS

EXERCISE	SET	1	2	3	4	5	6
	REPS						
	WEIGHT						
	REPS						
	WEIGHT						
	REPS						
	WEIGHT						
	REPS						
	WEIGHT						
	REPS						
	WEIGHT						
	REPS						
	WEIGHT						
	REPS						
	WEIGHT						
	REPS						
	WEIGHT						
	REPS						
	WEIGHT						
	REPS						
	WEIGHT						

CARDIO	TIME	DISTANCE	HEART RATE	CALS BURNED

MEASUREMENTS

NECK	
R BICEP	
L BICEP	
CHEST	
WAIST	
HIPS	
R THIGH	
L THIGH	
CALF	

NOTES/NUTUITION

DATE: _____ ☐ ☐ ☐ ☐ ☐ ☐ ☐   WEIGHT: _____
           S M T W T F S

MUSCLE GROUP: _____ START TIME: _____ FINISH TIME: _____

STRENGTH TRAINING   HOW I FEEL: 😀 😊 😐 😠 😣   WATER: 8oz 8oz 8oz 8oz 8oz 8oz 8oz

☐ UPPER BODY   ☐ LOWER BODY   ☐ ABS

EXERCISE	SET	1	2	3	4	5	6
	REPS						
	WEIGHT						
	REPS						
	WEIGHT						
	REPS						
	WEIGHT						
	REPS						
	WEIGHT						
	REPS						
	WEIGHT						
	REPS						
	WEIGHT						
	REPS						
	WEIGHT						
	REPS						
	WEIGHT						
	REPS						
	WEIGHT						
	REPS						
	WEIGHT						

CARDIO	TIME	DISTANCE	HEART RATE	CALS BURNED

MEASUREMENTS

NECK	
R BICEP	
L BICEP	
CHEST	
WAIST	
HIPS	
R THIGH	
L THIGH	
CALF	

NOTES/NUTUITION

DATE: _____ ☐S ☐M ☐T ☐W ☐T ☐F ☐S   WEIGHT: _____

MUSCLE GROUP: _____ START TIME: _____ FINISH TIME: _____

STRENGTH TRAINING   HOW I FEEL: 😊 😌 😕 😣 😠   WATER: 8oz 8oz 8oz 8oz 8oz 8oz 8oz 8oz

☐ UPPER BODY   ☐ LOWER BODY   ☐ ABS

EXERCISE	SET	1	2	3	4	5	6
	REPS						
	WEIGHT						
	REPS						
	WEIGHT						
	REPS						
	WEIGHT						
	REPS						
	WEIGHT						
	REPS						
	WEIGHT						
	REPS						
	WEIGHT						
	REPS						
	WEIGHT						
	REPS						
	WEIGHT						
	REPS						
	WEIGHT						
	REPS						
	WEIGHT						

CARDIO	TIME	DISTANCE	HEART RATE	CALS BURNED

MEASUREMENTS

NECK	
R BICEP	
L BICEP	
CHEST	
WAIST	
HIPS	
R THIGH	
L THIGH	
CALF	

NOTES/NUTUITION

DATE: _____   □ □ □ □ □ □ □   WEIGHT: _____
                        S M T W T F S

MUSCLE GROUP: _____ START TIME: _____ FINISH TIME: _____

STRENGTH TRAINING   HOW I FEEL: 😊 🙂 😐 😒 😠   WATER: 8oz. 8oz. 8oz. 8oz. 8oz. 8oz. 8oz. 8oz.

□ UPPER BODY   □ LOWER BODY   □ ABS

EXERCISE	SET	1	2	3	4	5	6
	REPS						
	WEIGHT						
	REPS						
	WEIGHT						
	REPS						
	WEIGHT						
	REPS						
	WEIGHT						
	REPS						
	WEIGHT						
	REPS						
	WEIGHT						
	REPS						
	WEIGHT						
	REPS						
	WEIGHT						
	REPS						
	WEIGHT						
	REPS						
	WEIGHT						

CARDIO	TIME	DISTANCE	HEART RATE	CALS BURNED

MEASUREMENTS

NECK	
R BICEP	
L BICEP	
CHEST	
WAIST	
HIPS	
R THIGH	
L THIGH	
CALF	

NOTES/NUTUITION

DATE: _____ S M T W T F S WEIGHT: _____

MUSCLE GROUP: _____ START TIME: _____ FINISH TIME: _____

STRENGTH TRAINING   HOW I FEEL: 😊 🙂 😐 😒 😣   WATER: 8oz. 8oz. 8oz. 8oz. 8oz. 8oz. 8oz. 8oz.

☐ UPPER BODY   ☐ LOWER BODY   ☐ ABS

EXERCISE	SET	1	2	3	4	5	6
	REPS						
	WEIGHT						
	REPS						
	WEIGHT						
	REPS						
	WEIGHT						
	REPS						
	WEIGHT						
	REPS						
	WEIGHT						
	REPS						
	WEIGHT						
	REPS						
	WEIGHT						
	REPS						
	WEIGHT						
	REPS						
	WEIGHT						
	REPS						
	WEIGHT						

CARDIO	TIME	DISTANCE	HEART RATE	CALS BURNED

MEASUREMENTS

NECK	
R BICEP	
L BICEP	
CHEST	
WAIST	
HIPS	
R THIGH	
L THIGH	
CALF	

NOTES/NUTUITION

DATE: _____ ☐ ☐ ☐ ☐ ☐ ☐ ☐   WEIGHT: _____
                                S M T W T F S

MUSCLE GROUP: _____ START TIME: _____ FINISH TIME: _____

STRENGTH TRAINING   HOW I FEEL: 😀 😊 😐 😒 😣   WATER: 8oz. 8oz. 8oz. 8oz. 8oz. 8oz. 8oz. 8oz.

☐ UPPER BODY   ☐ LOWER BODY   ☐ ABS

EXERCISE	SET	1	2	3	4	5	6
	REPS						
	WEIGHT						
	REPS						
	WEIGHT						
	REPS						
	WEIGHT						
	REPS						
	WEIGHT						
	REPS						
	WEIGHT						
	REPS						
	WEIGHT						
	REPS						
	WEIGHT						
	REPS						
	WEIGHT						
	REPS						
	WEIGHT						
	REPS						
	WEIGHT						

CARDIO	TIME	DISTANCE	HEART RATE	CALS BURNED

MEASUREMENTS

NECK	
R BICEP	
L BICEP	
CHEST	
WAIST	
HIPS	
R THIGH	
L THIGH	
CALF	

NOTES/NUTUITION

DATE: _____ S M T W T F S WEIGHT: _____

MUSCLE GROUP: _____ START TIME: _____ FINISH TIME: _____

STRENGTH TRAINING HOW I FEEL: 😀 😊 😐 😣 😫 WATER: 8 oz. 8 oz. 8 oz. 8 oz. 8 oz. 8 oz. 8 oz. 8 oz.

☐ UPPER BODY ☐ LOWER BODY ☐ ABS

EXERCISE	SET	1	2	3	4	5	6
	REPS						
	WEIGHT						
	REPS						
	WEIGHT						
	REPS						
	WEIGHT						
	REPS						
	WEIGHT						
	REPS						
	WEIGHT						
	REPS						
	WEIGHT						
	REPS						
	WEIGHT						
	REPS						
	WEIGHT						
	REPS						
	WEIGHT						
	REPS						
	WEIGHT						

CARDIO	TIME	DISTANCE	HEART RATE	CALS BURNED

NOTES/NUTUITION

MEASUREMENTS

NECK	
R BICEP	
L BICEP	
CHEST	
WAIST	
HIPS	
R THIGH	
L THIGH	
CALF	

DATE: _____ ☐ ☐ ☐ ☐ ☐ ☐ ☐   WEIGHT: _____
              S M T W T F S

MUSCLE GROUP: _____ START TIME: _____ FINISH TIME: _____

STRENGTH TRAINING   HOW I FEEL: 😃 😊 😐 😫 😠   WATER: 8oz. 8oz. 8oz. 8oz. 8oz. 8oz. 8oz. 8oz.

☐ UPPER BODY   ☐ LOWER BODY   ☐ ABS

EXERCISE	SET	1	2	3	4	5	6
	REPS						
	WEIGHT						
	REPS						
	WEIGHT						
	REPS						
	WEIGHT						
	REPS						
	WEIGHT						
	REPS						
	WEIGHT						
	REPS						
	WEIGHT						
	REPS						
	WEIGHT						
	REPS						
	WEIGHT						
	REPS						
	WEIGHT						
	REPS						
	WEIGHT						

CARDIO   TIME   DISTANCE   HEART RATE   CALS BURNED

MEASUREMENTS

NECK	
R BICEP	
L BICEP	
CHEST	
WAIST	
HIPS	
R THIGH	
L THIGH	
CALF	

NOTES/NUTUITION

DATE: _____ S M T W T F S WEIGHT: _____

MUSCLE GROUP: _____ START TIME: _____ FINISH TIME: _____

STRENGTH TRAINING HOW I FEEL: 😀 😊 😐 😣 😠 WATER: 8 oz. 8 oz. 8 oz. 8 oz. 8 oz. 8 oz. 8 oz. 8 oz.

☐ UPPER BODY ☐ LOWER BODY ☐ ABS

EXERCISE	SET	1	2	3	4	5	6
	REPS						
	WEIGHT						
	REPS						
	WEIGHT						
	REPS						
	WEIGHT						
	REPS						
	WEIGHT						
	REPS						
	WEIGHT						
	REPS						
	WEIGHT						
	REPS						
	WEIGHT						
	REPS						
	WEIGHT						
	REPS						
	WEIGHT						
	REPS						
	WEIGHT						

CARDIO	TIME	DISTANCE	HEART RATE	CALS BURNED

MEASUREMENTS

NECK	
R BICEP	
L BICEP	
CHEST	
WAIST	
HIPS	
R THIGH	
L THIGH	
CALF	

NOTES/NUTUITION

DATE: _____ ☐ ☐ ☐ ☐ ☐ ☐ ☐   WEIGHT: _____
                                 S M T W T F S

MUSCLE GROUP: _____ START TIME: _____ FINISH TIME: _____

STRENGTH TRAINING   HOW I FEEL: 😀 😊 😐 😟 😣   WATER: 8oz 8oz 8oz 8oz 8oz 8oz 8oz 8oz

☐ UPPER BODY   ☐ LOWER BODY   ☐ ABS

EXERCISE	SET	1	2	3	4	5	6
	REPS						
	WEIGHT						
	REPS						
	WEIGHT						
	REPS						
	WEIGHT						
	REPS						
	WEIGHT						
	REPS						
	WEIGHT						
	REPS						
	WEIGHT						
	REPS						
	WEIGHT						
	REPS						
	WEIGHT						
	REPS						
	WEIGHT						
	REPS						
	WEIGHT						

CARDIO	TIME	DISTANCE	HEART RATE	CALS BURNED

MEASUREMENTS

NECK	
R BICEP	
L BICEP	
CHEST	
WAIST	
HIPS	
R THIGH	
L THIGH	
CALF	

NOTES/NUTUITION

DATE: _____ ☐ ☐ ☐ ☐ ☐ ☐ ☐   WEIGHT: _____
           S M T W T F S

MUSCLE GROUP: _____   START TIME: _____   FINISH TIME: _____

STRENGTH TRAINING   HOW I FEEL: 😊 😌 😐 😕 😠   WATER: 8oz 8oz 8oz 8oz 8oz 8oz 8oz 8oz

☐ UPPER BODY   ☐ LOWER BODY   ☐ ABS

EXERCISE	SET	1	2	3	4	5	6
	REPS						
	WEIGHT						
	REPS						
	WEIGHT						
	REPS						
	WEIGHT						
	REPS						
	WEIGHT						
	REPS						
	WEIGHT						
	REPS						
	WEIGHT						
	REPS						
	WEIGHT						
	REPS						
	WEIGHT						
	REPS						
	WEIGHT						
	REPS						
	WEIGHT						

CARDIO   TIME   DISTANCE   HEART RATE   CALS BURNED

MEASUREMENTS

NECK	
R BICEP	
L BICEP	
CHEST	
WAIST	
HIPS	
R THIGH	
L THIGH	
CALF	

NOTES/NUTUITION

DATE: _____ S M T W T F S WEIGHT: _____

MUSCLE GROUP: _____ START TIME: _____ FINISH TIME: _____

STRENGTH TRAINING   HOW I FEEL: 😀 😊 😐 😒 😠   WATER: 8oz 8oz 8oz 8oz 8oz 8oz 8oz 8oz

| ☐ UPPER BODY | ☐ LOWER BODY | ☐ ABS |

EXERCISE	SET	1	2	3	4	5	6
	REPS						
	WEIGHT						
	REPS						
	WEIGHT						
	REPS						
	WEIGHT						
	REPS						
	WEIGHT						
	REPS						
	WEIGHT						
	REPS						
	WEIGHT						
	REPS						
	WEIGHT						
	REPS						
	WEIGHT						
	REPS						
	WEIGHT						
	REPS						
	WEIGHT						

CARDIO	TIME	DISTANCE	HEART RATE	CALS BURNED

MEASUREMENTS

NECK	
R BICEP	
L BICEP	
CHEST	
WAIST	
HIPS	
R THIGH	
L THIGH	
CALF	

NOTES/NUTUITION

DATE: _____ ☐ ☐ ☐ ☐ ☐ ☐ ☐   WEIGHT: _____
               S M T W T F S

MUSCLE GROUP: _____ START TIME: _____ FINISH TIME: _____

STRENGTH TRAINING   HOW I FEEL: 😊 🙂 😐 😒 😣   WATER: ☐ ☐ ☐ ☐ ☐ ☐ ☐ ☐
                                                         8oz 8oz 8oz 8oz 8oz 8oz 8oz 8oz

☐ UPPER BODY   ☐ LOWER BODY   ☐ ABS

EXERCISE	SET	1	2	3	4	5	6
	REPS						
	WEIGHT						
	REPS						
	WEIGHT						
	REPS						
	WEIGHT						
	REPS						
	WEIGHT						
	REPS						
	WEIGHT						
	REPS						
	WEIGHT						
	REPS						
	WEIGHT						
	REPS						
	WEIGHT						
	REPS						
	WEIGHT						
	REPS						
	WEIGHT						

CARDIO	TIME	DISTANCE	HEART RATE	CALS BURNED

MEASUREMENTS

NECK	
R BICEP	
L BICEP	
CHEST	
WAIST	
HIPS	
R THIGH	
L THIGH	
CALF	

NOTES/NUTUITION

DATE: _____ ☐☐☐☐☐☐☐ WEIGHT: _____
                                S M T W T F S

MUSCLE GROUP: _____ START TIME: _____ FINISH TIME: _____

STRENGTH TRAINING   HOW I FEEL: 😀 😊 😐 😖 😠   WATER: 8oz 8oz 8oz 8oz 8oz 8oz 8oz 8oz

☐ UPPER BODY   ☐ LOWER BODY   ☐ ABS

EXERCISE	SET	1	2	3	4	5	6
	REPS						
	WEIGHT						
	REPS						
	WEIGHT						
	REPS						
	WEIGHT						
	REPS						
	WEIGHT						
	REPS						
	WEIGHT						
	REPS						
	WEIGHT						
	REPS						
	WEIGHT						
	REPS						
	WEIGHT						
	REPS						
	WEIGHT						
	REPS						
	WEIGHT						

CARDIO	TIME	DISTANCE	HEART RATE	CALS BURNED

MEASUREMENTS

NECK	
R BICEP	
L BICEP	
CHEST	
WAIST	
HIPS	
R THIGH	
L THIGH	
CALF	

NOTES/NUTUITION

DATE: _____ ☐S ☐M ☐T ☐W ☐T ☐F ☐S   WEIGHT: _____

MUSCLE GROUP: _____ START TIME: _____ FINISH TIME: _____

STRENGTH TRAINING   HOW I FEEL: 😊 🙂 😐 😣 😠   WATER: ☐8oz ☐8oz ☐8oz ☐8oz ☐8oz ☐8oz ☐8oz ☐8oz

☐ UPPER BODY   ☐ LOWER BODY   ☐ ABS

EXERCISE	SET	1	2	3	4	5	6
	REPS						
	WEIGHT						
	REPS						
	WEIGHT						
	REPS						
	WEIGHT						
	REPS						
	WEIGHT						
	REPS						
	WEIGHT						
	REPS						
	WEIGHT						
	REPS						
	WEIGHT						
	REPS						
	WEIGHT						
	REPS						
	WEIGHT						
	REPS						
	WEIGHT						

CARDIO	TIME	DISTANCE	HEART RATE	CALS BURNED

MEASUREMENTS

NECK	
R BICEP	
L BICEP	
CHEST	
WAIST	
HIPS	
R THIGH	
L THIGH	
CALF	

NOTES/NUTUITION

DATE: _____ S M T W T F S WEIGHT: _____

MUSCLE GROUP: _____ START TIME: _____ FINISH TIME: _____

STRENGTH TRAINING HOW I FEEL: 😀 😊 😐 😫 😡 WATER: 8 oz. 8 oz. 8 oz. 8 oz. 8 oz. 8 oz. 8 oz. 8 oz.

- [ ] UPPER BODY
- [ ] LOWER BODY
- [ ] ABS

EXERCISE	SET	1	2	3	4	5	6
	REPS						
	WEIGHT						
	REPS						
	WEIGHT						
	REPS						
	WEIGHT						
	REPS						
	WEIGHT						
	REPS						
	WEIGHT						
	REPS						
	WEIGHT						
	REPS						
	WEIGHT						
	REPS						
	WEIGHT						
	REPS						
	WEIGHT						
	REPS						
	WEIGHT						

CARDIO	TIME	DISTANCE	HEART RATE	CALS BURNED

MEASUREMENTS

NECK	
R BICEP	
L BICEP	
CHEST	
WAIST	
HIPS	
R THIGH	
L THIGH	
CALF	

NOTES/NUTUITION

DATE: _____ S M T W T F S   WEIGHT: _____

MUSCLE GROUP: _____ START TIME: _____ FINISH TIME: _____

STRENGTH TRAINING HOW I FEEL: 😊 🙂 😐 😣 😤 WATER: 8oz. 8oz. 8oz. 8oz. 8oz. 8oz. 8oz. 8oz.

☐ UPPER BODY ☐ LOWER BODY ☐ ABS

EXERCISE	SET	1	2	3	4	5	6
	REPS						
	WEIGHT						
	REPS						
	WEIGHT						
	REPS						
	WEIGHT						
	REPS						
	WEIGHT						
	REPS						
	WEIGHT						
	REPS						
	WEIGHT						
	REPS						
	WEIGHT						
	REPS						
	WEIGHT						
	REPS						
	WEIGHT						
	REPS						
	WEIGHT						

CARDIO	TIME	DISTANCE	HEART RATE	CALS BURNED

MEASUREMENTS

NECK	
R BICEP	
L BICEP	
CHEST	
WAIST	
HIPS	
R THIGH	
L THIGH	
CALF	

NOTES/NUTUITION

DATE: _____ S M T W T F S   WEIGHT: _____

MUSCLE GROUP: _____ START TIME: _____ FINISH TIME: _____

STRENGTH TRAINING   HOW I FEEL: 😊 🙂 😐 🤢 😣   WATER: 8oz 8oz 8oz 8oz 8oz 8oz 8oz 8oz

- [ ] UPPER BODY
- [ ] LOWER BODY
- [ ] ABS

EXERCISE	SET	1	2	3	4	5	6
	REPS						
	WEIGHT						
	REPS						
	WEIGHT						
	REPS						
	WEIGHT						
	REPS						
	WEIGHT						
	REPS						
	WEIGHT						
	REPS						
	WEIGHT						
	REPS						
	WEIGHT						
	REPS						
	WEIGHT						
	REPS						
	WEIGHT						
	REPS						
	WEIGHT						

CARDIO	TIME	DISTANCE	HEART RATE	CALS BURNED

MEASUREMENTS

NECK	
R BICEP	
L BICEP	
CHEST	
WAIST	
HIPS	
R THIGH	
L THIGH	
CALF	

NOTES/NUTUITION

DATE: _____ S M T W T F S WEIGHT: _____

MUSCLE GROUP: _____ START TIME: _____ FINISH TIME: _____

STRENGTH TRAINING HOW I FEEL: 😀 😊 😐 😒 😖 WATER: 8 oz. 8 oz. 8 oz. 8 oz. 8 oz. 8 oz. 8 oz. 8 oz.

☐ UPPER BODY ☐ LOWER BODY ☐ ABS

EXERCISE	SET	1	2	3	4	5	6
	REPS						
	WEIGHT						
	REPS						
	WEIGHT						
	REPS						
	WEIGHT						
	REPS						
	WEIGHT						
	REPS						
	WEIGHT						
	REPS						
	WEIGHT						
	REPS						
	WEIGHT						
	REPS						
	WEIGHT						
	REPS						
	WEIGHT						
	REPS						
	WEIGHT						

CARDIO	TIME	DISTANCE	HEART RATE	CALS BURNED

MEASUREMENTS

NECK	
R BICEP	
L BICEP	
CHEST	
WAIST	
HIPS	
R THIGH	
L THIGH	
CALF	

NOTES/NUTUITION

DATE: _____ ☐ ☐ ☐ ☐ ☐ ☐ ☐   WEIGHT: _____
               S M T W T F S

MUSCLE GROUP: _____ START TIME: _____ FINISH TIME: _____

STRENGTH TRAINING   HOW I FEEL: 😊 😌 😐 😖 😣   WATER: 8oz 8oz 8oz 8oz 8oz 8oz 8oz 8oz

☐ UPPER BODY   ☐ LOWER BODY   ☐ ABS

EXERCISE	SET	1	2	3	4	5	6
	REPS						
	WEIGHT						
	REPS						
	WEIGHT						
	REPS						
	WEIGHT						
	REPS						
	WEIGHT						
	REPS						
	WEIGHT						
	REPS						
	WEIGHT						
	REPS						
	WEIGHT						
	REPS						
	WEIGHT						
	REPS						
	WEIGHT						
	REPS						
	WEIGHT						

CARDIO	TIME	DISTANCE	HEART RATE	CALS BURNED

MEASUREMENTS

NECK	
R BICEP	
L BICEP	
CHEST	
WAIST	
HIPS	
R THIGH	
L THIGH	
CALF	

NOTES/NUTUITION

DATE: _____ S M T W T F S WEIGHT: _____

MUSCLE GROUP: _____ START TIME: _____ FINISH TIME: _____

STRENGTH TRAINING   HOW I FEEL: 😀 🙂 😐 😣 😠   WATER: 8 oz. 8 oz. 8 oz. 8 oz. 8 oz. 8 oz. 8 oz. 8 oz.

☐ UPPER BODY   ☐ LOWER BODY   ☐ ABS

EXERCISE	SET	1	2	3	4	5	6
	REPS						
	WEIGHT						
	REPS						
	WEIGHT						
	REPS						
	WEIGHT						
	REPS						
	WEIGHT						
	REPS						
	WEIGHT						
	REPS						
	WEIGHT						
	REPS						
	WEIGHT						
	REPS						
	WEIGHT						
	REPS						
	WEIGHT						
	REPS						
	WEIGHT						

CARDIO	TIME	DISTANCE	HEART RATE	CALS BURNED

MEASUREMENTS

NECK	
R BICEP	
L BICEP	
CHEST	
WAIST	
HIPS	
R THIGH	
L THIGH	
CALF	

NOTES/NUTUITION

DATE: _____ ☐ ☐ ☐ ☐ ☐ ☐ WEIGHT: _____
　　　　　　　　　　　　　　　　S M T W T F S

MUSCLE GROUP: _____ START TIME: _____ FINISH TIME: _____

STRENGTH TRAINING   HOW I FEEL: 😊 😄 😐 😖 😠   WATER: 8oz 8oz 8oz 8oz 8oz 8oz 8oz 8oz

☐ UPPER BODY　　　　　☐ LOWER BODY　　　　　☐ ABS

EXERCISE	SET	1	2	3	4	5	6
	REPS						
	WEIGHT						
	REPS						
	WEIGHT						
	REPS						
	WEIGHT						
	REPS						
	WEIGHT						
	REPS						
	WEIGHT						
	REPS						
	WEIGHT						
	REPS						
	WEIGHT						
	REPS						
	WEIGHT						
	REPS						
	WEIGHT						
	REPS						
	WEIGHT						

CARDIO	TIME	DISTANCE	HEART RATE	CALS BURNED

MEASUREMENTS

NECK	
R BICEP	
L BICEP	
CHEST	
WAIST	
HIPS	
R THIGH	
L THIGH	
CALF	

NOTES/NUTUITION

DATE: _____ ☐S ☐M ☐T ☐W ☐T ☐F ☐S   WEIGHT: _____

MUSCLE GROUP: _____ START TIME: _____ FINISH TIME: _____

STRENGTH TRAINING   HOW I FEEL: 😀 😊 😐 😞 😠   WATER: ☐8oz ☐8oz ☐8oz ☐8oz ☐8oz ☐8oz ☐8oz ☐8oz

☐ UPPER BODY   ☐ LOWER BODY   ☐ ABS

EXERCISE	SET	1	2	3	4	5	6
	REPS						
	WEIGHT						
	REPS						
	WEIGHT						
	REPS						
	WEIGHT						
	REPS						
	WEIGHT						
	REPS						
	WEIGHT						
	REPS						
	WEIGHT						
	REPS						
	WEIGHT						
	REPS						
	WEIGHT						
	REPS						
	WEIGHT						
	REPS						
	WEIGHT						

CARDIO	TIME	DISTANCE	HEART RATE	CALS BURNED

MEASUREMENTS

NECK	
R BICEP	
L BICEP	
CHEST	
WAIST	
HIPS	
R THIGH	
L THIGH	
CALF	

NOTES/NUTUITION

DATE: _____ ☐ ☐ ☐ ☐ ☐ ☐ ☐   WEIGHT: _____
                                 S M T W T F S

MUSCLE GROUP: _____ START TIME: _____ FINISH TIME: _____

STRENGTH TRAINING   HOW I FEEL: 😀 😊 😐 😒 😣   WATER: 8oz 8oz 8oz 8oz 8oz 8oz 8oz 8oz

| ☐ UPPER BODY | ☐ LOWER BODY | ☐ ABS |

EXERCISE	SET	1	2	3	4	5	6
	REPS						
	WEIGHT						
	REPS						
	WEIGHT						
	REPS						
	WEIGHT						
	REPS						
	WEIGHT						
	REPS						
	WEIGHT						
	REPS						
	WEIGHT						
	REPS						
	WEIGHT						
	REPS						
	WEIGHT						
	REPS						
	WEIGHT						
	REPS						
	WEIGHT						

CARDIO	TIME	DISTANCE	HEART RATE	CALS BURNED

MEASUREMENTS

NECK	
R BICEP	
L BICEP	
CHEST	
WAIST	
HIPS	
R THIGH	
L THIGH	
CALF	

NOTES/NUTUITION

DATE: _____ S M T W T F S WEIGHT: _____

MUSCLE GROUP: _____ START TIME: _____ FINISH TIME: _____

STRENGTH TRAINING HOW I FEEL: 😊 😐 😕 😫 😣 WATER: 8oz. 8oz. 8oz. 8oz. 8oz. 8oz. 8oz. 8oz.

☐ UPPER BODY ☐ LOWER BODY ☐ ABS

EXERCISE	SET	1	2	3	4	5	6
	REPS						
	WEIGHT						
	REPS						
	WEIGHT						
	REPS						
	WEIGHT						
	REPS						
	WEIGHT						
	REPS						
	WEIGHT						
	REPS						
	WEIGHT						
	REPS						
	WEIGHT						
	REPS						
	WEIGHT						
	REPS						
	WEIGHT						
	REPS						
	WEIGHT						

CARDIO	TIME	DISTANCE	HEART RATE	CALS BURNED

MEASUREMENTS

NECK	
R BICEP	
L BICEP	
CHEST	
WAIST	
HIPS	
R THIGH	
L THIGH	
CALF	

NOTES/NUTUITION

DATE: _____ ☐ ☐ ☐ ☐ ☐ ☐ ☐   WEIGHT: _____
                              S M T W T F S

MUSCLE GROUP: _____ START TIME: _____ FINISH TIME: _____

STRENGTH TRAINING   HOW I FEEL: 😀 😊 😐 😖 😠   WATER: 8oz 8oz 8oz 8oz 8oz 8oz 8oz 8oz

☐ UPPER BODY   ☐ LOWER BODY   ☐ ABS

EXERCISE	SET	1	2	3	4	5	6
	REPS						
	WEIGHT						
	REPS						
	WEIGHT						
	REPS						
	WEIGHT						
	REPS						
	WEIGHT						
	REPS						
	WEIGHT						
	REPS						
	WEIGHT						
	REPS						
	WEIGHT						
	REPS						
	WEIGHT						
	REPS						
	WEIGHT						
	REPS						
	WEIGHT						

CARDIO	TIME	DISTANCE	HEART RATE	CALS BURNED

MEASUREMENTS

NECK	
R BICEP	
L BICEP	
CHEST	
WAIST	
HIPS	
R THIGH	
L THIGH	
CALF	

NOTES/NUTUITION

DATE: _____ S M T W T F S WEIGHT: _____

MUSCLE GROUP: _____ START TIME: _____ FINISH TIME: _____

STRENGTH TRAINING   HOW I FEEL: 😀 😊 😐 😒 😠   WATER: 8oz 8oz 8oz 8oz 8oz 8oz 8oz 8oz

☐ UPPER BODY   ☐ LOWER BODY   ☐ ABS

EXERCISE	SET	1	2	3	4	5	6
	REPS						
	WEIGHT						
	REPS						
	WEIGHT						
	REPS						
	WEIGHT						
	REPS						
	WEIGHT						
	REPS						
	WEIGHT						
	REPS						
	WEIGHT						
	REPS						
	WEIGHT						
	REPS						
	WEIGHT						
	REPS						
	WEIGHT						
	REPS						
	WEIGHT						

CARDIO	TIME	DISTANCE	HEART RATE	CALS BURNED

MEASUREMENTS

NECK	
R BICEP	
L BICEP	
CHEST	
WAIST	
HIPS	
R THIGH	
L THIGH	
CALF	

NOTES/NUTUITION

DATE: _____ ☐ ☐ ☐ ☐ ☐ ☐ ☐   WEIGHT: _____
                                 S M T W T F S

MUSCLE GROUP: _____ START TIME: _____ FINISH TIME: _____

STRENGTH TRAINING   HOW I FEEL: 😀 😊 😐 😒 😣   WATER: 8oz. 8oz. 8oz. 8oz. 8oz. 8oz. 8oz. 8oz. 8oz.

☐ UPPER BODY   ☐ LOWER BODY   ☐ ABS

EXERCISE	SET	1	2	3	4	5	6
	REPS						
	WEIGHT						
	REPS						
	WEIGHT						
	REPS						
	WEIGHT						
	REPS						
	WEIGHT						
	REPS						
	WEIGHT						
	REPS						
	WEIGHT						
	REPS						
	WEIGHT						
	REPS						
	WEIGHT						
	REPS						
	WEIGHT						
	REPS						
	WEIGHT						

CARDIO	TIME	DISTANCE	HEART RATE	CALS BURNED

MEASUREMENTS

NECK	
R BICEP	
L BICEP	
CHEST	
WAIST	
HIPS	
R THIGH	
L THIGH	
CALF	

NOTES/NUTRITION

DATE: _____ S M T W T F S WEIGHT: _____

MUSCLE GROUP: _____ START TIME: _____ FINISH TIME: _____

STRENGTH TRAINING HOW I FEEL: 😊 🙂 😐 😣 😠 WATER: 8 oz. 8 oz. 8 oz. 8 oz. 8 oz. 8 oz. 8 oz. 8 oz.

☐ UPPER BODY ☐ LOWER BODY ☐ ABS

EXERCISE	SET	1	2	3	4	5	6
	REPS						
	WEIGHT						
	REPS						
	WEIGHT						
	REPS						
	WEIGHT						
	REPS						
	WEIGHT						
	REPS						
	WEIGHT						
	REPS						
	WEIGHT						
	REPS						
	WEIGHT						
	REPS						
	WEIGHT						
	REPS						
	WEIGHT						
	REPS						
	WEIGHT						

CARDIO	TIME	DISTANCE	HEART RATE	CALS BURNED

MEASUREMENTS

NECK	
R BICEP	
L BICEP	
CHEST	
WAIST	
HIPS	
R THIGH	
L THIGH	
CALF	

NOTES/NUTUITION

DATE: _____ S M T W T F S WEIGHT: _____

MUSCLE GROUP: _____ START TIME: _____ FINISH TIME: _____

STRENGTH TRAINING HOW I FEEL: 😀 🙂 😐 😣 😖 WATER: 8oz 8oz 8oz 8oz 8oz 8oz 8oz 8oz

☐ UPPER BODY ☐ LOWER BODY ☐ ABS

EXERCISE	SET	1	2	3	4	5	6
	REPS						
	WEIGHT						
	REPS						
	WEIGHT						
	REPS						
	WEIGHT						
	REPS						
	WEIGHT						
	REPS						
	WEIGHT						
	REPS						
	WEIGHT						
	REPS						
	WEIGHT						
	REPS						
	WEIGHT						
	REPS						
	WEIGHT						
	REPS						
	WEIGHT						

CARDIO	TIME	DISTANCE	HEART RATE	CALS BURNED

MEASUREMENTS

NECK	
R BICEP	
L BICEP	
CHEST	
WAIST	
HIPS	
R THIGH	
L THIGH	
CALF	

NOTES/NUTUITION

DATE: _____ □ □ □ □ □ □ WEIGHT: _____
                                S M T W T F S

MUSCLE GROUP: _____ START TIME: _____ FINISH TIME: _____

STRENGTH TRAINING   HOW I FEEL: 😀 😊 😐 😣 😠   WATER: ○ ○ ○ ○ ○ ○ ○ ○
                                                        oz. oz. oz. oz. oz. oz. oz. oz.

| ☐ UPPER BODY | ☐ LOWER BODY | ☐ ABS |

EXERCISE	SET	1	2	3	4	5	6
	REPS						
	WEIGHT						
	REPS						
	WEIGHT						
	REPS						
	WEIGHT						
	REPS						
	WEIGHT						
	REPS						
	WEIGHT						
	REPS						
	WEIGHT						
	REPS						
	WEIGHT						
	REPS						
	WEIGHT						
	REPS						
	WEIGHT						
	REPS						
	WEIGHT						

CARDIO	TIME	DISTANCE	HEART RATE	CALS BURNED

MEASUREMENTS

NECK	
R BICEP	
L BICEP	
CHEST	
WAIST	
HIPS	
R THIGH	
L THIGH	
CALF	

NOTES/NUTUITION

DATE: _____ ☐ ☐ ☐ ☐ ☐ ☐ ☐   WEIGHT: _____
                                S M T W T F S

MUSCLE GROUP: _____ START TIME: _____ FINISH TIME: _____

STRENGTH TRAINING   HOW I FEEL: 😀 😊 😐 🤢 😣   WATER: 8oz 8oz 8oz 8oz 8oz 8oz 8oz 8oz

☐ UPPER BODY   ☐ LOWER BODY   ☐ ABS

EXERCISE	SET	1	2	3	4	5	6
	REPS						
	WEIGHT						
	REPS						
	WEIGHT						
	REPS						
	WEIGHT						
	REPS						
	WEIGHT						
	REPS						
	WEIGHT						
	REPS						
	WEIGHT						
	REPS						
	WEIGHT						
	REPS						
	WEIGHT						
	REPS						
	WEIGHT						
	REPS						
	WEIGHT						

CARDIO	TIME	DISTANCE	HEART RATE	CALS BURNED

MEASUREMENTS

NECK	
R BICEP	
L BICEP	
CHEST	
WAIST	
HIPS	
R THIGH	
L THIGH	
CALF	

NOTES/NUTUITION

DATE: _____ S M T W T F S WEIGHT: _____

MUSCLE GROUP: _____ START TIME: _____ FINISH TIME: _____

STRENGTH TRAINING HOW I FEEL: 😊 🙂 😐 😫 😣 WATER: 8oz 8oz 8oz 8oz 8oz 8oz 8oz 8oz 8oz

☐ UPPER BODY   ☐ LOWER BODY   ☐ ABS

EXERCISE	SET	1	2	3	4	5	6
	REPS						
	WEIGHT						
	REPS						
	WEIGHT						
	REPS						
	WEIGHT						
	REPS						
	WEIGHT						
	REPS						
	WEIGHT						
	REPS						
	WEIGHT						
	REPS						
	WEIGHT						
	REPS						
	WEIGHT						
	REPS						
	WEIGHT						
	REPS						
	WEIGHT						

CARDIO	TIME	DISTANCE	HEART RATE	CALS BURNED

MEASUREMENTS

NECK	
R BICEP	
L BICEP	
CHEST	
WAIST	
HIPS	
R THIGH	
L THIGH	
CALF	

NOTES/NUTUITION

DATE: _____ ☐ ☐ ☐ ☐ ☐ ☐ ☐   WEIGHT: _____
                              S M T W T F S

MUSCLE GROUP: _____   START TIME: _____   FINISH TIME: _____

STRENGTH TRAINING   HOW I FEEL: 😀 😊 😐 😣 😠   WATER: 8oz. 8oz. 8oz. 8oz. 8oz. 8oz. 8oz. 8oz.

☐ UPPER BODY   ☐ LOWER BODY   ☐ ABS

EXERCISE	SET	1	2	3	4	5	6
	REPS						
	WEIGHT						
	REPS						
	WEIGHT						
	REPS						
	WEIGHT						
	REPS						
	WEIGHT						
	REPS						
	WEIGHT						
	REPS						
	WEIGHT						
	REPS						
	WEIGHT						
	REPS						
	WEIGHT						
	REPS						
	WEIGHT						
	REPS						
	WEIGHT						

CARDIO	TIME	DISTANCE	HEART RATE	CALS BURNED

MEASUREMENTS

NECK	
R BICEP	
L BICEP	
CHEST	
WAIST	
HIPS	
R THIGH	
L THIGH	
CALF	

NOTES/NUTUITION

DATE: _____ S M T W T F S WEIGHT: _____

MUSCLE GROUP: _____ START TIME: _____ FINISH TIME: _____

STRENGTH TRAINING HOW I FEEL: 😊 😐 😶 😟 😠 WATER: 8 oz. 8 oz. 8 oz. 8 oz. 8 oz. 8 oz. 8 oz. 8 oz.

☐ UPPER BODY ☐ LOWER BODY ☐ ABS

EXERCISE	SET	1	2	3	4	5	6
	REPS						
	WEIGHT						
	REPS						
	WEIGHT						
	REPS						
	WEIGHT						
	REPS						
	WEIGHT						
	REPS						
	WEIGHT						
	REPS						
	WEIGHT						
	REPS						
	WEIGHT						
	REPS						
	WEIGHT						
	REPS						
	WEIGHT						
	REPS						
	WEIGHT						

CARDIO	TIME	DISTANCE	HEART RATE	CALS BURNED

MEASUREMENTS

NECK	
R BICEP	
L BICEP	
CHEST	
WAIST	
HIPS	
R THIGH	
L THIGH	
CALF	

NOTES/NUTUITION

DATE: _____   S M T W T F S   WEIGHT: _____

MUSCLE GROUP: _____ START TIME: _____ FINISH TIME: _____

STRENGTH TRAINING   HOW I FEEL: 😀 😊 😐 😖 😠   WATER: 8oz 8oz 8oz 8oz 8oz 8oz 8oz 8oz 8oz

☐ UPPER BODY	☐ LOWER BODY	☐ ABS

EXERCISE	SET	1	2	3	4	5	6
	REPS						
	WEIGHT						
	REPS						
	WEIGHT						
	REPS						
	WEIGHT						
	REPS						
	WEIGHT						
	REPS						
	WEIGHT						
	REPS						
	WEIGHT						
	REPS						
	WEIGHT						
	REPS						
	WEIGHT						
	REPS						
	WEIGHT						
	REPS						
	WEIGHT						

CARDIO	TIME	DISTANCE	HEART RATE	CALS BURNED

MEASUREMENTS

NECK	
R BICEP	
L BICEP	
CHEST	
WAIST	
HIPS	
R THIGH	
L THIGH	
CALF	

NOTES/NUTUITION

DATE: _____ S M T W T F S WEIGHT: _____

MUSCLE GROUP: _____ START TIME: _____ FINISH TIME: _____

STRENGTH TRAINING   HOW I FEEL: 😊 😌 😐 😣 😠   WATER: 8oz 8oz 8oz 8oz 8oz 8oz 8oz 8oz

☐ UPPER BODY   ☐ LOWER BODY   ☐ ABS

EXERCISE	SET	1	2	3	4	5	6
	REPS						
	WEIGHT						
	REPS						
	WEIGHT						
	REPS						
	WEIGHT						
	REPS						
	WEIGHT						
	REPS						
	WEIGHT						
	REPS						
	WEIGHT						
	REPS						
	WEIGHT						
	REPS						
	WEIGHT						
	REPS						
	WEIGHT						
	REPS						
	WEIGHT						

CARDIO	TIME	DISTANCE	HEART RATE	CALS BURNED

MEASUREMENTS

NECK	
R BICEP	
L BICEP	
CHEST	
WAIST	
HIPS	
R THIGH	
L THIGH	
CALF	

NOTES/NUTUITION

DATE: _____   ☐S ☐M ☐T ☐W ☐T ☐F ☐S   WEIGHT: _____

MUSCLE GROUP: _____   START TIME: _____   FINISH TIME: _____

STRENGTH TRAINING   HOW I FEEL: 😀 😊 😐 😖 😠   WATER: 8oz 8oz 8oz 8oz 8oz 8oz 8oz 8oz

☐ UPPER BODY   ☐ LOWER BODY   ☐ ABS

EXERCISE	SET	1	2	3	4	5	6
	REPS						
	WEIGHT						
	REPS						
	WEIGHT						
	REPS						
	WEIGHT						
	REPS						
	WEIGHT						
	REPS						
	WEIGHT						
	REPS						
	WEIGHT						
	REPS						
	WEIGHT						
	REPS						
	WEIGHT						
	REPS						
	WEIGHT						
	REPS						
	WEIGHT						

CARDIO	TIME	DISTANCE	HEART RATE	CALS BURNED

MEASUREMENTS

NECK	
R BICEP	
L BICEP	
CHEST	
WAIST	
HIPS	
R THIGH	
L THIGH	
CALF	

NOTES/NUTUITION

DATE: _____ S M T W T F S WEIGHT: _____

MUSCLE GROUP: _____ START TIME: _____ FINISH TIME: _____

STRENGTH TRAINING HOW I FEEL: 😊 🙂 😐 😒 😠 WATER: 8oz. 8oz. 8oz. 8oz. 8oz. 8oz. 8oz. 8oz.

- [ ] UPPER BODY
- [ ] LOWER BODY
- [ ] ABS

EXERCISE	SET	1	2	3	4	5	6
	REPS						
	WEIGHT						
	REPS						
	WEIGHT						
	REPS						
	WEIGHT						
	REPS						
	WEIGHT						
	REPS						
	WEIGHT						
	REPS						
	WEIGHT						
	REPS						
	WEIGHT						
	REPS						
	WEIGHT						
	REPS						
	WEIGHT						
	REPS						
	WEIGHT						

CARDIO	TIME	DISTANCE	HEART RATE	CALS BURNED

MEASUREMENTS

NECK	
R BICEP	
L BICEP	
CHEST	
WAIST	
HIPS	
R THIGH	
L THIGH	
CALF	

NOTES/NUTUITION

DATE: _____ ☐ ☐ ☐ ☐ ☐ ☐ ☐   WEIGHT: _____
             S M T W T F S

MUSCLE GROUP: _____ START TIME: _____ FINISH TIME: _____

STRENGTH TRAINING   HOW I FEEL: 😀 😊 😐 😣 😠   WATER: 8oz 8oz 8oz 8oz 8oz 8oz 8oz 8oz

☐ UPPER BODY   ☐ LOWER BODY   ☐ ABS

EXERCISE	SET	1	2	3	4	5	6
	REPS						
	WEIGHT						
	REPS						
	WEIGHT						
	REPS						
	WEIGHT						
	REPS						
	WEIGHT						
	REPS						
	WEIGHT						
	REPS						
	WEIGHT						
	REPS						
	WEIGHT						
	REPS						
	WEIGHT						
	REPS						
	WEIGHT						
	REPS						
	WEIGHT						

CARDIO   TIME   DISTANCE   HEART RATE   CALS BURNED   MEASUREMENTS

NECK	
R BICEP	
L BICEP	
CHEST	
WAIST	
HIPS	
R THIGH	
L THIGH	
CALF	

NOTES/NUTUITION

DATE: _____ S M T W T F S WEIGHT: _____

MUSCLE GROUP: _____ START TIME: _____ FINISH TIME: _____

STRENGTH TRAINING HOW I FEEL: 😀 😊 😐 😠 😡 WATER: 8 oz. 8 oz. 8 oz. 8 oz. 8 oz. 8 oz. 8 oz. 8 oz.

☐ UPPER BODY ☐ LOWER BODY ☐ ABS

EXERCISE	SET	1	2	3	4	5	6
	REPS						
	WEIGHT						
	REPS						
	WEIGHT						
	REPS						
	WEIGHT						
	REPS						
	WEIGHT						
	REPS						
	WEIGHT						
	REPS						
	WEIGHT						
	REPS						
	WEIGHT						
	REPS						
	WEIGHT						
	REPS						
	WEIGHT						
	REPS						
	WEIGHT						

CARDIO	TIME	DISTANCE	HEART RATE	CALS BURNED

MEASUREMENTS

NECK	
R BICEP	
L BICEP	
CHEST	
WAIST	
HIPS	
R THIGH	
L THIGH	
CALF	

NOTES/NUTUITION

DATE: _____ ☐S ☐M ☐T ☐W ☐T ☐F ☐S   WEIGHT: _____

MUSCLE GROUP: _____ START TIME: _____ FINISH TIME: _____

STRENGTH TRAINING   HOW I FEEL: 😀 😊 😐 😣 😫   WATER: 8oz. 8oz. 8oz. 8oz. 8oz. 8oz. 8oz. 8oz.

☐ UPPER BODY   ☐ LOWER BODY   ☐ ABS

EXERCISE	SET	1	2	3	4	5	6
	REPS						
	WEIGHT						
	REPS						
	WEIGHT						
	REPS						
	WEIGHT						
	REPS						
	WEIGHT						
	REPS						
	WEIGHT						
	REPS						
	WEIGHT						
	REPS						
	WEIGHT						
	REPS						
	WEIGHT						
	REPS						
	WEIGHT						
	REPS						
	WEIGHT						

CARDIO	TIME	DISTANCE	HEART RATE	CALS BURNED

MEASUREMENTS	
NECK	
R BICEP	
L BICEP	
CHEST	
WAIST	
HIPS	
R THIGH	
L THIGH	
CALF	

NOTES/NUTUITION

DATE: _____ S M T W T F S WEIGHT: _____

MUSCLE GROUP: _____ START TIME: _____ FINISH TIME: _____

STRENGTH TRAINING HOW I FEEL: 😊 😌 😐 😠 😣 WATER: 8oz 8oz 8oz 8oz 8oz 8oz 8oz 8oz

- [ ] UPPER BODY
- [ ] LOWER BODY
- [ ] ABS

EXERCISE	SET	1	2	3	4	5	6
	REPS						
	WEIGHT						
	REPS						
	WEIGHT						
	REPS						
	WEIGHT						
	REPS						
	WEIGHT						
	REPS						
	WEIGHT						
	REPS						
	WEIGHT						
	REPS						
	WEIGHT						
	REPS						
	WEIGHT						
	REPS						
	WEIGHT						
	REPS						
	WEIGHT						

CARDIO	TIME	DISTANCE	HEART RATE	CALS BURNED

NOTES/NUTUITION

MEASUREMENTS

NECK	
R BICEP	
L BICEP	
CHEST	
WAIST	
HIPS	
R THIGH	
L THIGH	
CALF	

DATE: _____ ☐ ☐ ☐ ☐ ☐ ☐ ☐   WEIGHT: _____
               S M T W T F S

MUSCLE GROUP: _____ START TIME: _____ FINISH TIME: _____

STRENGTH TRAINING   HOW I FEEL: 😀 😉 😐 😣 😠   WATER: 8oz 8oz 8oz 8oz 8oz 8oz 8oz 8oz

☐ UPPER BODY   ☐ LOWER BODY   ☐ ABS

EXERCISE	SET	1	2	3	4	5	6
	REPS						
	WEIGHT						
	REPS						
	WEIGHT						
	REPS						
	WEIGHT						
	REPS						
	WEIGHT						
	REPS						
	WEIGHT						
	REPS						
	WEIGHT						
	REPS						
	WEIGHT						
	REPS						
	WEIGHT						
	REPS						
	WEIGHT						
	REPS						
	WEIGHT						

CARDIO	TIME	DISTANCE	HEART RATE	CALS BURNED

MEASUREMENTS

NECK	
R BICEP	
L BICEP	
CHEST	
WAIST	
HIPS	
R THIGH	
L THIGH	
CALF	

NOTES/NUTUITION

DATE: _____ □ □ □ □ □ □ □   WEIGHT: _____
                          S M T W T F S

MUSCLE GROUP: _____ START TIME: _____ FINISH TIME: _____

STRENGTH TRAINING   HOW I FEEL: 😊 🙂 😐 😕 😠   WATER: 8oz. 8oz. 8oz. 8oz. 8oz. 8oz. 8oz. 8oz.

□ UPPER BODY   □ LOWER BODY   □ ABS

EXERCISE	SET	1	2	3	4	5	6
	REPS						
	WEIGHT						
	REPS						
	WEIGHT						
	REPS						
	WEIGHT						
	REPS						
	WEIGHT						
	REPS						
	WEIGHT						
	REPS						
	WEIGHT						
	REPS						
	WEIGHT						
	REPS						
	WEIGHT						
	REPS						
	WEIGHT						
	REPS						
	WEIGHT						

CARDIO	TIME	DISTANCE	HEART RATE	CALS BURNED

MEASUREMENTS

NECK	
R BICEP	
L BICEP	
CHEST	
WAIST	
HIPS	
R THIGH	
L THIGH	
CALF	

NOTES/NUTUITION

DATE: _____ S M T W T F S   WEIGHT: _____

MUSCLE GROUP: _____ START TIME: _____ FINISH TIME: _____

STRENGTH TRAINING   HOW I FEEL: 😀 😊 😐 😖 😣   WATER: 8oz 8oz 8oz 8oz 8oz 8oz 8oz 8oz

☐ UPPER BODY   ☐ LOWER BODY   ☐ ABS

EXERCISE	SET	1	2	3	4	5	6
	REPS						
	WEIGHT						
	REPS						
	WEIGHT						
	REPS						
	WEIGHT						
	REPS						
	WEIGHT						
	REPS						
	WEIGHT						
	REPS						
	WEIGHT						
	REPS						
	WEIGHT						
	REPS						
	WEIGHT						
	REPS						
	WEIGHT						
	REPS						
	WEIGHT						

CARDIO	TIME	DISTANCE	HEART RATE	CALS BURNED

MEASUREMENTS

NECK	
R BICEP	
L BICEP	
CHEST	
WAIST	
HIPS	
R THIGH	
L THIGH	
CALF	

NOTES/NUTUITION

DATE: _____ ☐S ☐M ☐T ☐W ☐T ☐F ☐S   WEIGHT: _____

MUSCLE GROUP: _____ START TIME: _____ FINISH TIME: _____

STRENGTH TRAINING   HOW I FEEL: 😀 😊 😐 😞 😣   WATER: ☐8oz. ☐8oz. ☐8oz. ☐8oz. ☐8oz. ☐8oz. ☐8oz. ☐8oz.

☐ UPPER BODY   ☐ LOWER BODY   ☐ ABS

EXERCISE	SET	1	2	3	4	5	6
	REPS						
	WEIGHT						
	REPS						
	WEIGHT						
	REPS						
	WEIGHT						
	REPS						
	WEIGHT						
	REPS						
	WEIGHT						
	REPS						
	WEIGHT						
	REPS						
	WEIGHT						
	REPS						
	WEIGHT						
	REPS						
	WEIGHT						
	REPS						
	WEIGHT						

CARDIO	TIME	DISTANCE	HEART RATE	CALS BURNED

MEASUREMENTS

NECK	
R BICEP	
L BICEP	
CHEST	
WAIST	
HIPS	
R THIGH	
L THIGH	
CALF	

NOTES/NUTUITION

DATE: _____ ☐ ☐ ☐ ☐ ☐ ☐ ☐ WEIGHT: _____
         S M T W T F S

MUSCLE GROUP: _____ START TIME: _____ FINISH TIME: _____

STRENGTH TRAINING   HOW I FEEL: 😀 😊 😐 😖 😠   WATER: 8oz 8oz 8oz 8oz 8oz 8oz 8oz 8oz

☐ UPPER BODY   ☐ LOWER BODY   ☐ ABS

EXERCISE	SET	1	2	3	4	5	6
	REPS						
	WEIGHT						
	REPS						
	WEIGHT						
	REPS						
	WEIGHT						
	REPS						
	WEIGHT						
	REPS						
	WEIGHT						
	REPS						
	WEIGHT						
	REPS						
	WEIGHT						
	REPS						
	WEIGHT						
	REPS						
	WEIGHT						
	REPS						
	WEIGHT						

CARDIO	TIME	DISTANCE	HEART RATE	CALS BURNED

MEASUREMENTS

NECK	
R BICEP	
L BICEP	
CHEST	
WAIST	
HIPS	
R THIGH	
L THIGH	
CALF	

NOTES/NUTUITION

DATE: _____ S M T W T F S WEIGHT: _____

MUSCLE GROUP: _____ START TIME: _____ FINISH TIME: _____

STRENGTH TRAINING   HOW I FEEL: 😊 🙂 😐 😣 😤   WATER: 8oz 8oz 8oz 8oz 8oz 8oz 8oz 8oz

- [ ] UPPER BODY
- [ ] LOWER BODY
- [ ] ABS

EXERCISE	SET	1	2	3	4	5	6
	REPS						
	WEIGHT						
	REPS						
	WEIGHT						
	REPS						
	WEIGHT						
	REPS						
	WEIGHT						
	REPS						
	WEIGHT						
	REPS						
	WEIGHT						
	REPS						
	WEIGHT						
	REPS						
	WEIGHT						
	REPS						
	WEIGHT						
	REPS						
	WEIGHT						

CARDIO	TIME	DISTANCE	HEART RATE	CALS BURNED

MEASUREMENTS

NECK	
R BICEP	
L BICEP	
CHEST	
WAIST	
HIPS	
R THIGH	
L THIGH	
CALF	

NOTES/NUTUITION

DATE: _____ S M T W T F S WEIGHT: _____

MUSCLE GROUP: _____ START TIME: _____ FINISH TIME: _____

STRENGTH TRAINING HOW I FEEL: 😀 😊 😐 😕 😠 WATER: 8oz 8oz 8oz 8oz 8oz 8oz 8oz 8oz

☐ UPPER BODY ☐ LOWER BODY ☐ ABS

EXERCISE	SET	1	2	3	4	5	6
	REPS						
	WEIGHT						
	REPS						
	WEIGHT						
	REPS						
	WEIGHT						
	REPS						
	WEIGHT						
	REPS						
	WEIGHT						
	REPS						
	WEIGHT						
	REPS						
	WEIGHT						
	REPS						
	WEIGHT						
	REPS						
	WEIGHT						
	REPS						
	WEIGHT						

CARDIO	TIME	DISTANCE	HEART RATE	CALS BURNED

MEASUREMENTS

NECK	
R BICEP	
L BICEP	
CHEST	
WAIST	
HIPS	
R THIGH	
L THIGH	
CALF	

NOTES/NUTUITION

DATE: _____ S M T W T F S   WEIGHT: _____

MUSCLE GROUP: _____ START TIME: _____ FINISH TIME: _____

STRENGTH TRAINING   HOW I FEEL: 😊 😌 😐 😟 😣   WATER: 8oz 8oz 8oz 8oz 8oz 8oz 8oz 8oz

- [ ] UPPER BODY
- [ ] LOWER BODY
- [ ] ABS

EXERCISE	SET	1	2	3	4	5	6
	REPS						
	WEIGHT						
	REPS						
	WEIGHT						
	REPS						
	WEIGHT						
	REPS						
	WEIGHT						
	REPS						
	WEIGHT						
	REPS						
	WEIGHT						
	REPS						
	WEIGHT						
	REPS						
	WEIGHT						
	REPS						
	WEIGHT						
	REPS						
	WEIGHT						

CARDIO	TIME	DISTANCE	HEART RATE	CALS BURNED

MEASUREMENTS

NECK	
R BICEP	
L BICEP	
CHEST	
WAIST	
HIPS	
R THIGH	
L THIGH	
CALF	

NOTES/NUTUITION

DATE: _____ ☐ ☐ ☐ ☐ ☐ ☐ ☐   WEIGHT: _____
                              S M T W T F S

MUSCLE GROUP: _____ START TIME: _____ FINISH TIME: _____

STRENGTH TRAINING   HOW I FEEL: 😀 😊 😐 😒 😠   WATER: 8oz. 8oz. 8oz. 8oz. 8oz. 8oz. 8oz. 8oz.

☐ UPPER BODY   ☐ LOWER BODY   ☐ ABS

EXERCISE	SET	1	2	3	4	5	6
	REPS						
	WEIGHT						
	REPS						
	WEIGHT						
	REPS						
	WEIGHT						
	REPS						
	WEIGHT						
	REPS						
	WEIGHT						
	REPS						
	WEIGHT						
	REPS						
	WEIGHT						
	REPS						
	WEIGHT						
	REPS						
	WEIGHT						
	REPS						
	WEIGHT						

CARDIO   TIME   DISTANCE   HEART RATE   CALS BURNED

MEASUREMENTS

NECK	
R BICEP	
L BICEP	
CHEST	
WAIST	
HIPS	
R THIGH	
L THIGH	
CALF	

NOTES/NUTUITION

DATE: _____ □S □M □T □W □T □F □S   WEIGHT: _____

MUSCLE GROUP: _____ START TIME: _____ FINISH TIME: _____

STRENGTH TRAINING   HOW I FEEL: 😀 🙂 😐 😣 😠   WATER: 8oz. 8oz. 8oz. 8oz. 8oz. 8oz. 8oz. 8oz.

□ UPPER BODY   □ LOWER BODY   □ ABS

EXERCISE	SET	1	2	3	4	5	6
	REPS						
	WEIGHT						
	REPS						
	WEIGHT						
	REPS						
	WEIGHT						
	REPS						
	WEIGHT						
	REPS						
	WEIGHT						
	REPS						
	WEIGHT						
	REPS						
	WEIGHT						
	REPS						
	WEIGHT						
	REPS						
	WEIGHT						
	REPS						
	WEIGHT						

CARDIO	TIME	DISTANCE	HEART RATE	CALS BURNED

MEASUREMENTS

NECK	
R BICEP	
L BICEP	
CHEST	
WAIST	
HIPS	
R THIGH	
L THIGH	
CALF	

NOTES/NUTUITION

DATE: _____ S M T W T F S WEIGHT: _____

MUSCLE GROUP: _____ START TIME: _____ FINISH TIME: _____

STRENGTH TRAINING HOW I FEEL: 😊 😌 😐 😣 😠 WATER: 8oz 8oz 8oz 8oz 8oz 8oz 8oz 8oz

☐ UPPER BODY   ☐ LOWER BODY   ☐ ABS

EXERCISE	SET	1	2	3	4	5	6
	REPS						
	WEIGHT						
	REPS						
	WEIGHT						
	REPS						
	WEIGHT						
	REPS						
	WEIGHT						
	REPS						
	WEIGHT						
	REPS						
	WEIGHT						
	REPS						
	WEIGHT						
	REPS						
	WEIGHT						
	REPS						
	WEIGHT						
	REPS						
	WEIGHT						

CARDIO	TIME	DISTANCE	HEART RATE	CALS BURNED

MEASUREMENTS

NECK	
R BICEP	
L BICEP	
CHEST	
WAIST	
HIPS	
R THIGH	
L THIGH	
CALF	

NOTES/NUTUITION

DATE: _____ ☐ ☐ ☐ ☐ ☐ ☐ ☐ WEIGHT: _____
                                S M T W T F S

MUSCLE GROUP: _____ START TIME: _____ FINISH TIME: _____

STRENGTH TRAINING   HOW I FEEL: 😊 😌 😐 😣 😤   WATER: 8oz. 8oz. 8oz. 8oz. 8oz. 8oz. 8oz. 8oz.

☐ UPPER BODY   ☐ LOWER BODY   ☐ ABS

EXERCISE	SET	1	2	3	4	5	6
	REPS						
	WEIGHT						
	REPS						
	WEIGHT						
	REPS						
	WEIGHT						
	REPS						
	WEIGHT						
	REPS						
	WEIGHT						
	REPS						
	WEIGHT						
	REPS						
	WEIGHT						
	REPS						
	WEIGHT						
	REPS						
	WEIGHT						
	REPS						
	WEIGHT						

CARDIO	TIME	DISTANCE	HEART RATE	CALS BURNED

MEASUREMENTS

NECK	
R BICEP	
L BICEP	
CHEST	
WAIST	
HIPS	
R THIGH	
L THIGH	
CALF	

NOTES/NUTUITION

DATE: _____ ☐☐☐☐☐☐☐ WEIGHT: _____
             S M T W T F S

MUSCLE GROUP: _____ START TIME: _____ FINISH TIME: _____

STRENGTH TRAINING   HOW I FEEL: 😀 😊 😐 😖 😠   WATER: 8oz 8oz 8oz 8oz 8oz 8oz 8oz 8oz

☐ UPPER BODY   ☐ LOWER BODY   ☐ ABS

EXERCISE	SET	1	2	3	4	5	6
	REPS						
	WEIGHT						
	REPS						
	WEIGHT						
	REPS						
	WEIGHT						
	REPS						
	WEIGHT						
	REPS						
	WEIGHT						
	REPS						
	WEIGHT						
	REPS						
	WEIGHT						
	REPS						
	WEIGHT						
	REPS						
	WEIGHT						
	REPS						
	WEIGHT						

CARDIO	TIME	DISTANCE	HEART RATE	CALS BURNED

MEASUREMENTS

NECK	
R BICEP	
L BICEP	
CHEST	
WAIST	
HIPS	
R THIGH	
L THIGH	
CALF	

NOTES/NUTUITION

DATE: _____ S M T W T F S WEIGHT: _____

MUSCLE GROUP: _____ START TIME: _____ FINISH TIME: _____

STRENGTH TRAINING HOW I FEEL: 😊 😐 😕 😣 WATER: 8oz 8oz 8oz 8oz 8oz 8oz 8oz 8oz

☐ UPPER BODY ☐ LOWER BODY ☐ ABS

EXERCISE	SET	1	2	3	4	5	6
	REPS						
	WEIGHT						
	REPS						
	WEIGHT						
	REPS						
	WEIGHT						
	REPS						
	WEIGHT						
	REPS						
	WEIGHT						
	REPS						
	WEIGHT						
	REPS						
	WEIGHT						
	REPS						
	WEIGHT						
	REPS						
	WEIGHT						
	REPS						
	WEIGHT						

CARDIO	TIME	DISTANCE	HEART RATE	CALS BURNED

MEASUREMENTS

NECK	
R BICEP	
L BICEP	
CHEST	
WAIST	
HIPS	
R THIGH	
L THIGH	
CALF	

NOTES/NUTUITION

DATE: _____ S M T W T F S   WEIGHT: _____

MUSCLE GROUP: _____ START TIME: _____ FINISH TIME: _____

STRENGTH TRAINING   HOW I FEEL: 😀 😊 😐 😣 😖   WATER: 8oz 8oz 8oz 8oz 8oz 8oz 8oz 8oz

- [ ] UPPER BODY
- [ ] LOWER BODY
- [ ] ABS

EXERCISE	SET	1	2	3	4	5	6
	REPS						
	WEIGHT						
	REPS						
	WEIGHT						
	REPS						
	WEIGHT						
	REPS						
	WEIGHT						
	REPS						
	WEIGHT						
	REPS						
	WEIGHT						
	REPS						
	WEIGHT						
	REPS						
	WEIGHT						
	REPS						
	WEIGHT						
	REPS						
	WEIGHT						

CARDIO	TIME	DISTANCE	HEART RATE	CALS BURNED

MEASUREMENTS

NECK	
R BICEP	
L BICEP	
CHEST	
WAIST	
HIPS	
R THIGH	
L THIGH	
CALF	

NOTES/NUTUITION

DATE: _____   ☐ ☐ ☐ ☐ ☐ ☐ ☐   WEIGHT: _____
                                 S M T W T F S

MUSCLE GROUP: _____ START TIME: _____ FINISH TIME: _____

STRENGTH TRAINING   HOW I FEEL: 😀 😊 😐 😣 😠   WATER: 2oz. 3oz. 4oz. 6oz. 8oz. 8oz. 8oz. 8oz. 8oz.

☐ UPPER BODY	☐ LOWER BODY	☐ ABS

EXERCISE	SET	1	2	3	4	5	6
	REPS						
	WEIGHT						
	REPS						
	WEIGHT						
	REPS						
	WEIGHT						
	REPS						
	WEIGHT						
	REPS						
	WEIGHT						
	REPS						
	WEIGHT						
	REPS						
	WEIGHT						
	REPS						
	WEIGHT						
	REPS						
	WEIGHT						
	REPS						
	WEIGHT						

CARDIO	TIME	DISTANCE	HEART RATE	CALS BURNED

MEASUREMENTS

NECK	
R BICEP	
L BICEP	
CHEST	
WAIST	
HIPS	
R THIGH	
L THIGH	
CALF	

NOTES/NUTUITION

DATE: _____ ☐ ☐ ☐ ☐ ☐ ☐ ☐   WEIGHT: _____
              S M T W T F S

MUSCLE GROUP: _____ START TIME: _____ FINISH TIME: _____

STRENGTH TRAINING   HOW I FEEL: 😊 😌 😐 😖 😠   WATER: 8oz. 8oz. 8oz. 8oz. 8oz. 8oz. 8oz. 8oz. 8oz.

☐ UPPER BODY   ☐ LOWER BODY   ☐ ABS

EXERCISE	SET	1	2	3	4	5	6
	REPS						
	WEIGHT						
	REPS						
	WEIGHT						
	REPS						
	WEIGHT						
	REPS						
	WEIGHT						
	REPS						
	WEIGHT						
	REPS						
	WEIGHT						
	REPS						
	WEIGHT						
	REPS						
	WEIGHT						
	REPS						
	WEIGHT						
	REPS						
	WEIGHT						

CARDIO	TIME	DISTANCE	HEART RATE	CALS BURNED

MEASUREMENTS

NECK	
R BICEP	
L BICEP	
CHEST	
WAIST	
HIPS	
R THIGH	
L THIGH	
CALF	

NOTES/NUTUITION

DATE: _____   ☐ ☐ ☐ ☐ ☐ ☐ ☐   WEIGHT: _____
                                 S M T W T F S

MUSCLE GROUP: _____ START TIME: _____ FINISH TIME: _____

STRENGTH TRAINING   HOW I FEEL: 😀 😊 😐 😒 😣   WATER: 8oz. 8oz. 8oz. 8oz. 8oz. 8oz. 8oz. 8oz.

☐ UPPER BODY   ☐ LOWER BODY   ☐ ABS

EXERCISE	SET	1	2	3	4	5	6
	REPS						
	WEIGHT						
	REPS						
	WEIGHT						
	REPS						
	WEIGHT						
	REPS						
	WEIGHT						
	REPS						
	WEIGHT						
	REPS						
	WEIGHT						
	REPS						
	WEIGHT						
	REPS						
	WEIGHT						
	REPS						
	WEIGHT						
	REPS						
	WEIGHT						

CARDIO	TIME	DISTANCE	HEART RATE	CALS BURNED

MEASUREMENTS

NECK	
R BICEP	
L BICEP	
CHEST	
WAIST	
HIPS	
R THIGH	
L THIGH	
CALF	

NOTES/NUTUITION

DATE: _____ ☐ ☐ ☐ ☐ ☐ ☐ ☐ WEIGHT: _____
                              S M T W T F S

MUSCLE GROUP: _____ START TIME: _____ FINISH TIME: _____

STRENGTH TRAINING HOW I FEEL: 😀 🙂 😐 😣 😠   WATER: 8oz 8oz 8oz 8oz 8oz 8oz 8oz 8oz

☐ UPPER BODY   ☐ LOWER BODY   ☐ ABS

EXERCISE	SET	1	2	3	4	5	6
	REPS						
	WEIGHT						
	REPS						
	WEIGHT						
	REPS						
	WEIGHT						
	REPS						
	WEIGHT						
	REPS						
	WEIGHT						
	REPS						
	WEIGHT						
	REPS						
	WEIGHT						
	REPS						
	WEIGHT						
	REPS						
	WEIGHT						
	REPS						
	WEIGHT						

CARDIO TIME DISTANCE HEART RATE CALS BURNED

MEASUREMENTS

NECK	
R BICEP	
L BICEP	
CHEST	
WAIST	
HIPS	
R THIGH	
L THIGH	
CALF	

NOTES/NUTUITION

DATE: _____ S M T W T F S WEIGHT: _____

MUSCLE GROUP: _____ START TIME: _____ FINISH TIME: _____

STRENGTH TRAINING HOW I FEEL: 😀 🙂 😐 😒 😠 WATER: 8oz. 8oz. 8oz. 8oz. 8oz. 8oz. 8oz. 8oz.

☐ UPPER BODY   ☐ LOWER BODY   ☐ ABS

EXERCISE	SET	1	2	3	4	5	6
	REPS						
	WEIGHT						
	REPS						
	WEIGHT						
	REPS						
	WEIGHT						
	REPS						
	WEIGHT						
	REPS						
	WEIGHT						
	REPS						
	WEIGHT						
	REPS						
	WEIGHT						
	REPS						
	WEIGHT						
	REPS						
	WEIGHT						
	REPS						
	WEIGHT						

CARDIO	TIME	DISTANCE	HEART RATE	CALS BURNED

MEASUREMENTS

NECK	
R BICEP	
L BICEP	
CHEST	
WAIST	
HIPS	
R THIGH	
L THIGH	
CALF	

NOTES/NUTUITION

DATE: _____ S M T W T F S   WEIGHT: _____

MUSCLE GROUP: _____ START TIME: _____ FINISH TIME: _____

STRENGTH TRAINING   HOW I FEEL: 😊 😌 😐 😫 😣   WATER: 8 oz. 8 oz. 8 oz. 8 oz. 8 oz. 8 oz. 8 oz. 8 oz.

☐ UPPER BODY   ☐ LOWER BODY   ☐ ABS

EXERCISE	SET	1	2	3	4	5	6
	REPS						
	WEIGHT						
	REPS						
	WEIGHT						
	REPS						
	WEIGHT						
	REPS						
	WEIGHT						
	REPS						
	WEIGHT						
	REPS						
	WEIGHT						
	REPS						
	WEIGHT						
	REPS						
	WEIGHT						
	REPS						
	WEIGHT						
	REPS						
	WEIGHT						

CARDIO	TIME	DISTANCE	HEART RATE	CALS BURNED

MEASUREMENTS

NECK	
R BICEP	
L BICEP	
CHEST	
WAIST	
HIPS	
R THIGH	
L THIGH	
CALF	

NOTES/NUTUITION

DATE: _____ 　□ □ □ □ □ □ □　WEIGHT: _____
　　　　　　　　　　　　　S M T W T F S

MUSCLE GROUP: _____ START TIME: _____ FINISH TIME: _____

STRENGTH TRAINING   HOW I FEEL: 😊 🙂 😐 😕 😠   WATER: 8oz. 8oz. 8oz. 8oz. 8oz. 8oz. 8oz. 8oz.

☐ UPPER BODY   ☐ LOWER BODY   ☐ ABS

EXERCISE	SET	1	2	3	4	5	6
	REPS						
	WEIGHT						
	REPS						
	WEIGHT						
	REPS						
	WEIGHT						
	REPS						
	WEIGHT						
	REPS						
	WEIGHT						
	REPS						
	WEIGHT						
	REPS						
	WEIGHT						
	REPS						
	WEIGHT						
	REPS						
	WEIGHT						
	REPS						
	WEIGHT						

CARDIO	TIME	DISTANCE	HEART RATE	CALS BURNED

MEASUREMENTS

NECK	
R BICEP	
L BICEP	
CHEST	
WAIST	
HIPS	
R THIGH	
L THIGH	
CALF	

NOTES/NUTUITION

DATE: _____   ☐ ☐ ☐ ☐ ☐ ☐   WEIGHT: _____
                                S M T W T F S

MUSCLE GROUP: _____   START TIME: _____   FINISH TIME: _____

STRENGTH TRAINING   HOW I FEEL: 😀 😊 😐 😒 😣   WATER: 8oz 8oz 8oz 8oz 8oz 8oz 8oz 8oz

☐ UPPER BODY   ☐ LOWER BODY   ☐ ABS

EXERCISE	SET	1	2	3	4	5	6
	REPS						
	WEIGHT						
	REPS						
	WEIGHT						
	REPS						
	WEIGHT						
	REPS						
	WEIGHT						
	REPS						
	WEIGHT						
	REPS						
	WEIGHT						
	REPS						
	WEIGHT						
	REPS						
	WEIGHT						
	REPS						
	WEIGHT						
	REPS						
	WEIGHT						

CARDIO	TIME	DISTANCE	HEART RATE	CALS BURNED

MEASUREMENTS

NECK	
R BICEP	
L BICEP	
CHEST	
WAIST	
HIPS	
R THIGH	
L THIGH	
CALF	

NOTES/NUTUITION

DATE: _____ S M T W T F S WEIGHT: _____

MUSCLE GROUP: _____ START TIME: _____ FINISH TIME: _____

STRENGTH TRAINING   HOW I FEEL: 😀 😊 😐 😖 😠   WATER: 8oz. 8oz. 8oz. 8oz. 8oz. 8oz. 8oz. 8oz.

☐ UPPER BODY   ☐ LOWER BODY   ☐ ABS

EXERCISE	SET	1	2	3	4	5	6
	REPS						
	WEIGHT						
	REPS						
	WEIGHT						
	REPS						
	WEIGHT						
	REPS						
	WEIGHT						
	REPS						
	WEIGHT						
	REPS						
	WEIGHT						
	REPS						
	WEIGHT						
	REPS						
	WEIGHT						
	REPS						
	WEIGHT						
	REPS						
	WEIGHT						

CARDIO	TIME	DISTANCE	HEART RATE	CALS BURNED

MEASUREMENTS

NECK	
R BICEP	
L BICEP	
CHEST	
WAIST	
HIPS	
R THIGH	
L THIGH	
CALF	

NOTES/NUTUITION

DATE: _____ ☐ ☐ ☐ ☐ ☐ ☐ ☐ WEIGHT: _____
                        S M T W T F S

MUSCLE GROUP: _____ START TIME: _____ FINISH TIME: _____

STRENGTH TRAINING   HOW I FEEL: 😊 😌 😐 😟 😣   WATER: 8oz. 8oz. 8oz. 8oz. 8oz. 8oz. 8oz. 8oz.

☐ UPPER BODY   ☐ LOWER BODY   ☐ ABS

EXERCISE	SET	1	2	3	4	5	6
	REPS						
	WEIGHT						
	REPS						
	WEIGHT						
	REPS						
	WEIGHT						
	REPS						
	WEIGHT						
	REPS						
	WEIGHT						
	REPS						
	WEIGHT						
	REPS						
	WEIGHT						
	REPS						
	WEIGHT						
	REPS						
	WEIGHT						
	REPS						
	WEIGHT						

CARDIO	TIME	DISTANCE	HEART RATE	CALS BURNED

MEASUREMENTS

NECK	
R BICEP	
L BICEP	
CHEST	
WAIST	
HIPS	
R THIGH	
L THIGH	
CALF	

NOTES/NUTUITION

DATE: _____ S M T W T F S WEIGHT: _____

MUSCLE GROUP: _____ START TIME: _____ FINISH TIME: _____

STRENGTH TRAINING   HOW I FEEL: 😀 😊 😐 😖 😠   WATER: 8oz 8oz 8oz 8oz 8oz 8oz 8oz 8oz

- [ ] UPPER BODY
- [ ] LOWER BODY
- [ ] ABS

EXERCISE	SET	1	2	3	4	5	6
	REPS						
	WEIGHT						
	REPS						
	WEIGHT						
	REPS						
	WEIGHT						
	REPS						
	WEIGHT						
	REPS						
	WEIGHT						
	REPS						
	WEIGHT						
	REPS						
	WEIGHT						
	REPS						
	WEIGHT						
	REPS						
	WEIGHT						
	REPS						
	WEIGHT						

CARDIO	TIME	DISTANCE	HEART RATE	CALS BURNED

MEASUREMENTS

NECK	
R BICEP	
L BICEP	
CHEST	
WAIST	
HIPS	
R THIGH	
L THIGH	
CALF	

NOTES/NUTUITION

DATE: _____ ☐ ☐ ☐ ☐ ☐ ☐ ☐   WEIGHT: _____
                                S M T W T F S

MUSCLE GROUP: _____ START TIME: _____ FINISH TIME: _____

STRENGTH TRAINING   HOW I FEEL: 😀 😊 😐 😕 😣   WATER: 8oz 8oz 8oz 8oz 8oz 8oz 8oz 8oz

☐ UPPER BODY   ☐ LOWER BODY   ☐ ABS

EXERCISE	SET	1	2	3	4	5	6
	REPS						
	WEIGHT						
	REPS						
	WEIGHT						
	REPS						
	WEIGHT						
	REPS						
	WEIGHT						
	REPS						
	WEIGHT						
	REPS						
	WEIGHT						
	REPS						
	WEIGHT						
	REPS						
	WEIGHT						
	REPS						
	WEIGHT						
	REPS						
	WEIGHT						

CARDIO	TIME	DISTANCE	HEART RATE	CALS BURNED

MEASUREMENTS

NECK	
R BICEP	
L BICEP	
CHEST	
WAIST	
HIPS	
R THIGH	
L THIGH	
CALF	

NOTES/NUTUITION

DATE: _____   S M T W T F S   WEIGHT: _____

MUSCLE GROUP: _____ START TIME: _____ FINISH TIME: _____

STRENGTH TRAINING   HOW I FEEL: 😀 😊 😐 😷 😣   WATER: 8oz. 8oz. 8oz. 8oz. 8oz. 8oz. 8oz. 8oz.

☐ UPPER BODY   ☐ LOWER BODY   ☐ ABS

EXERCISE	SET	1	2	3	4	5	6
	REPS						
	WEIGHT						
	REPS						
	WEIGHT						
	REPS						
	WEIGHT						
	REPS						
	WEIGHT						
	REPS						
	WEIGHT						
	REPS						
	WEIGHT						
	REPS						
	WEIGHT						
	REPS						
	WEIGHT						
	REPS						
	WEIGHT						
	REPS						
	WEIGHT						

CARDIO	TIME	DISTANCE	HEART RATE	CALS BURNED

MEASUREMENTS

NECK	
R BICEP	
L BICEP	
CHEST	
WAIST	
HIPS	
R THIGH	
L THIGH	
CALF	

NOTES/NUTUITION

DATE: _____ ☐ ☐ ☐ ☐ ☐ ☐ ☐   WEIGHT: _____
                       S M T W T F S

MUSCLE GROUP: _____ START TIME: _____ FINISH TIME: _____

STRENGTH TRAINING   HOW I FEEL: 😀 😊 😐 😒 😣   WATER: 8oz 8oz 8oz 8oz 8oz 8oz 8oz 8oz 8oz 8oz

☐ UPPER BODY   ☐ LOWER BODY   ☐ ABS

EXERCISE	SET	1	2	3	4	5	6
	REPS						
	WEIGHT						
	REPS						
	WEIGHT						
	REPS						
	WEIGHT						
	REPS						
	WEIGHT						
	REPS						
	WEIGHT						
	REPS						
	WEIGHT						
	REPS						
	WEIGHT						
	REPS						
	WEIGHT						
	REPS						
	WEIGHT						
	REPS						
	WEIGHT						

CARDIO	TIME	DISTANCE	HEART RATE	CALS BURNED

MEASUREMENTS

NECK	
R BICEP	
L BICEP	
CHEST	
WAIST	
HIPS	
R THIGH	
L THIGH	
CALF	

NOTES/NUTUITION

DATE: _____ ☐ ☐ ☐ ☐ ☐ ☐ ☐   WEIGHT: _____
                              S M T W T F S

MUSCLE GROUP: _____ START TIME: _____ FINISH TIME: _____

STRENGTH TRAINING   HOW I FEEL: 😀 😊 😐 😟 😣   WATER: 8oz 8oz 8oz 8oz 8oz 8oz 8oz 8oz

☐ UPPER BODY   ☐ LOWER BODY   ☐ ABS

EXERCISE	SET	1	2	3	4	5	6
	REPS						
	WEIGHT						
	REPS						
	WEIGHT						
	REPS						
	WEIGHT						
	REPS						
	WEIGHT						
	REPS						
	WEIGHT						
	REPS						
	WEIGHT						
	REPS						
	WEIGHT						
	REPS						
	WEIGHT						
	REPS						
	WEIGHT						
	REPS						
	WEIGHT						

CARDIO	TIME	DISTANCE	HEART RATE	CALS BURNED

MEASUREMENTS

NECK	
R BICEP	
L BICEP	
CHEST	
WAIST	
HIPS	
R THIGH	
L THIGH	
CALF	

NOTES/NUTUITION

DATE: _____ ☐ ☐ ☐ ☐ ☐ ☐ ☐ WEIGHT: _____
             S M T W T F S

MUSCLE GROUP: _____ START TIME: _____ FINISH TIME: _____

STRENGTH TRAINING   HOW I FEEL: 😀 😊 😐 😕 😣   WATER: 8oz 8oz 8oz 8oz 8oz 8oz 8oz 8oz

☐ UPPER BODY   ☐ LOWER BODY   ☐ ABS

EXERCISE	SET	1	2	3	4	5	6
	REPS						
	WEIGHT						
	REPS						
	WEIGHT						
	REPS						
	WEIGHT						
	REPS						
	WEIGHT						
	REPS						
	WEIGHT						
	REPS						
	WEIGHT						
	REPS						
	WEIGHT						
	REPS						
	WEIGHT						
	REPS						
	WEIGHT						
	REPS						
	WEIGHT						

CARDIO   TIME   DISTANCE   HEART RATE   CALS BURNED

MEASUREMENTS

NECK	
R BICEP	
L BICEP	
CHEST	
WAIST	
HIPS	
R THIGH	
L THIGH	
CALF	

NOTES/NUTUITION

DATE: _____ □ □ □ □ □ □ □   WEIGHT: _____
                        S M T W T F S

MUSCLE GROUP: _____   START TIME: _____   FINISH TIME: _____

STRENGTH TRAINING   HOW I FEEL: 😊 😄 😐 😕 😣   WATER: □ □ □ □ □ □ □ □
                                                       oz. oz. oz. oz. oz. oz. oz. oz.

□ UPPER BODY   □ LOWER BODY   □ ABS

EXERCISE	SET	1	2	3	4	5	6
	REPS						
	WEIGHT						
	REPS						
	WEIGHT						
	REPS						
	WEIGHT						
	REPS						
	WEIGHT						
	REPS						
	WEIGHT						
	REPS						
	WEIGHT						
	REPS						
	WEIGHT						
	REPS						
	WEIGHT						
	REPS						
	WEIGHT						
	REPS						
	WEIGHT						

CARDIO   TIME   DISTANCE   HEART RATE   CALS BURNED

MEASUREMENTS

NECK	
R BICEP	
L BICEP	
CHEST	
WAIST	
HIPS	
R THIGH	
L THIGH	
CALF	

NOTES/NUTUITION

DATE: _____ ☐ ☐ ☐ ☐ ☐ ☐ ☐   WEIGHT: _____
                                S M T W T F S

MUSCLE GROUP: _____ START TIME: _____ FINISH TIME: _____

STRENGTH TRAINING   HOW I FEEL: 😊 😌 😐 😠 😣   WATER: 8oz 8oz 8oz 8oz 8oz 8oz 8oz 8oz

☐ UPPER BODY   ☐ LOWER BODY   ☐ ABS

EXERCISE	SET	1	2	3	4	5	6
	REPS						
	WEIGHT						
	REPS						
	WEIGHT						
	REPS						
	WEIGHT						
	REPS						
	WEIGHT						
	REPS						
	WEIGHT						
	REPS						
	WEIGHT						
	REPS						
	WEIGHT						
	REPS						
	WEIGHT						
	REPS						
	WEIGHT						
	REPS						
	WEIGHT						

CARDIO	TIME	DISTANCE	HEART RATE	CALS BURNED

MEASUREMENTS

NECK	
R BICEP	
L BICEP	
CHEST	
WAIST	
HIPS	
R THIGH	
L THIGH	
CALF	

NOTES/NUTUITION

DATE: _____ ☐ ☐ ☐ ☐ ☐ ☐ ☐ WEIGHT: _____
                       S M T W T F S

MUSCLE GROUP: _____ START TIME: _____ FINISH TIME: _____

STRENGTH TRAINING   HOW I FEEL: 😊 😊 😐 😖 😣   WATER: 8oz. 8oz. 8oz. 8oz. 8oz. 8oz. 8oz. 8oz.

☐ UPPER BODY   ☐ LOWER BODY   ☐ ABS

EXERCISE	SET	1	2	3	4	5	6
	REPS						
	WEIGHT						
	REPS						
	WEIGHT						
	REPS						
	WEIGHT						
	REPS						
	WEIGHT						
	REPS						
	WEIGHT						
	REPS						
	WEIGHT						
	REPS						
	WEIGHT						
	REPS						
	WEIGHT						
	REPS						
	WEIGHT						
	REPS						
	WEIGHT						

CARDIO	TIME	DISTANCE	HEART RATE	CALS BURNED

MEASUREMENTS

NECK	
R BICEP	
L BICEP	
CHEST	
WAIST	
HIPS	
R THIGH	
L THIGH	
CALF	

NOTES/NUTUITION

DATE: _____   □ □ □ □ □ □ □   WEIGHT: _____
                                 S M T W T F S

MUSCLE GROUP: _____   START TIME: _____   FINISH TIME: _____

STRENGTH TRAINING   HOW I FEEL: 😀 😊 😐 😠 😣   WATER: 8oz 8oz 8oz 8oz 8oz 8oz 8oz 8oz

☐ UPPER BODY   ☐ LOWER BODY   ☐ ABS

EXERCISE	SET	1	2	3	4	5	6
	REPS						
	WEIGHT						
	REPS						
	WEIGHT						
	REPS						
	WEIGHT						
	REPS						
	WEIGHT						
	REPS						
	WEIGHT						
	REPS						
	WEIGHT						
	REPS						
	WEIGHT						
	REPS						
	WEIGHT						
	REPS						
	WEIGHT						
	REPS						
	WEIGHT						

CARDIO   TIME   DISTANCE   HEART RATE   CALS BURNED   MEASUREMENTS

CARDIO	TIME	DISTANCE	HEART RATE	CALS BURNED

MEASUREMENTS	
NECK	
R BICEP	
L BICEP	
CHEST	
WAIST	
HIPS	
R THIGH	
L THIGH	
CALF	

NOTES/NUTUITION

DATE: _____ ☐ ☐ ☐ ☐ ☐ ☐ ☐ WEIGHT: _____
                              S M T W T F S

MUSCLE GROUP: _____ START TIME: _____ FINISH TIME: _____

STRENGTH TRAINING   HOW I FEEL: 😃 🙂 😐 😟 😣   WATER: 8oz 8oz 8oz 8oz 8oz 8oz 8oz 8oz

☐ UPPER BODY   ☐ LOWER BODY   ☐ ABS

EXERCISE	SET	1	2	3	4	5	6
	REPS						
	WEIGHT						
	REPS						
	WEIGHT						
	REPS						
	WEIGHT						
	REPS						
	WEIGHT						
	REPS						
	WEIGHT						
	REPS						
	WEIGHT						
	REPS						
	WEIGHT						
	REPS						
	WEIGHT						
	REPS						
	WEIGHT						
	REPS						
	WEIGHT						

CARDIO	TIME	DISTANCE	HEART RATE	CALS BURNED

MEASUREMENTS

NECK	
R BICEP	
L BICEP	
CHEST	
WAIST	
HIPS	
R THIGH	
L THIGH	
CALF	

NOTES/NUTUITION

DATE: _____ S M T W T F S   WEIGHT: _____

MUSCLE GROUP: _____ START TIME: _____ FINISH TIME: _____

STRENGTH TRAINING   HOW I FEEL: 😀 😊 😐 😠 😫   WATER: 8 oz. 8 oz. 8 oz. 8 oz. 8 oz. 8 oz. 8 oz. 8 oz. 8 oz.

☐ UPPER BODY   ☐ LOWER BODY   ☐ ABS

EXERCISE	SET	1	2	3	4	5	6
	REPS						
	WEIGHT						
	REPS						
	WEIGHT						
	REPS						
	WEIGHT						
	REPS						
	WEIGHT						
	REPS						
	WEIGHT						
	REPS						
	WEIGHT						
	REPS						
	WEIGHT						
	REPS						
	WEIGHT						
	REPS						
	WEIGHT						
	REPS						
	WEIGHT						

CARDIO	TIME	DISTANCE	HEART RATE	CALS BURNED

MEASUREMENTS

NECK	
R BICEP	
L BICEP	
CHEST	
WAIST	
HIPS	
R THIGH	
L THIGH	
CALF	

NOTES/NUTUITION

DATE: _____ ☐ ☐ ☐ ☐ ☐ ☐ ☐ WEIGHT: _____
                                                               S M T W T F S

MUSCLE GROUP: _____ START TIME: _____ FINISH TIME: _____

STRENGTH TRAINING   HOW I FEEL: 😊 😄 😐 😟 😣   WATER: 8oz 8oz 8oz 8oz 8oz 8oz 8oz 8oz 8oz

☐ UPPER BODY   ☐ LOWER BODY   ☐ ABS

EXERCISE	SET	1	2	3	4	5	6
	REPS						
	WEIGHT						
	REPS						
	WEIGHT						
	REPS						
	WEIGHT						
	REPS						
	WEIGHT						
	REPS						
	WEIGHT						
	REPS						
	WEIGHT						
	REPS						
	WEIGHT						
	REPS						
	WEIGHT						
	REPS						
	WEIGHT						
	REPS						
	WEIGHT						

CARDIO	TIME	DISTANCE	HEART RATE	CALS BURNED

MEASUREMENTS

NECK	
R BICEP	
L BICEP	
CHEST	
WAIST	
HIPS	
R THIGH	
L THIGH	
CALF	

NOTES/NUTUITION

DATE: _____ S M T W T F S WEIGHT: _____

MUSCLE GROUP: _____ START TIME: _____ FINISH TIME: _____

STRENGTH TRAINING   HOW I FEEL: 😊 😌 😐 😣 😠   WATER: 8oz 8oz 8oz 8oz 8oz 8oz 8oz 8oz 8oz 8oz

☐ UPPER BODY   ☐ LOWER BODY   ☐ ABS

EXERCISE	SET	1	2	3	4	5	6
	REPS						
	WEIGHT						
	REPS						
	WEIGHT						
	REPS						
	WEIGHT						
	REPS						
	WEIGHT						
	REPS						
	WEIGHT						
	REPS						
	WEIGHT						
	REPS						
	WEIGHT						
	REPS						
	WEIGHT						
	REPS						
	WEIGHT						
	REPS						
	WEIGHT						

CARDIO   TIME   DISTANCE   HEART RATE   CALS BURNED

MEASUREMENTS

NECK	
R BICEP	
L BICEP	
CHEST	
WAIST	
HIPS	
R THIGH	
L THIGH	
CALF	

NOTES/NUTUITION

DATE: _____ □ □ □ □ □ □ □ WEIGHT: _____
             S M T W T F S

MUSCLE GROUP: _____ START TIME: _____ FINISH TIME: _____

STRENGTH TRAINING   HOW I FEEL: 😊 😄 😐 😕 😣   WATER: 8oz. 8oz. 8oz. 8oz. 8oz. 8oz. 8oz. 8oz.

□ UPPER BODY   □ LOWER BODY   □ ABS

EXERCISE	SET	1	2	3	4	5	6
	REPS						
	WEIGHT						
	REPS						
	WEIGHT						
	REPS						
	WEIGHT						
	REPS						
	WEIGHT						
	REPS						
	WEIGHT						
	REPS						
	WEIGHT						
	REPS						
	WEIGHT						
	REPS						
	WEIGHT						
	REPS						
	WEIGHT						
	REPS						
	WEIGHT						

CARDIO	TIME	DISTANCE	HEART RATE	CALS BURNED

MEASUREMENTS

NECK	
R BICEP	
L BICEP	
CHEST	
WAIST	
HIPS	
R THIGH	
L THIGH	
CALF	

NOTES/NUTUITION

DATE: _____ ☐ ☐ ☐ ☐ ☐ ☐ ☐   WEIGHT: _____
S M T W T F S

MUSCLE GROUP: _____ START TIME: _____ FINISH TIME: _____

STRENGTH TRAINING   HOW I FEEL: 😃 😊 😐 😒 😣   WATER: 8oz. 8oz. 8oz. 8oz. 8oz. 8oz. 8oz. 8oz.

☐ UPPER BODY ☐ LOWER BODY ☐ ABS

EXERCISE	SET	1	2	3	4	5	6
	REPS						
	WEIGHT						
	REPS						
	WEIGHT						
	REPS						
	WEIGHT						
	REPS						
	WEIGHT						
	REPS						
	WEIGHT						
	REPS						
	WEIGHT						
	REPS						
	WEIGHT						
	REPS						
	WEIGHT						
	REPS						
	WEIGHT						
	REPS						
	WEIGHT						

CARDIO   TIME   DISTANCE   HEART RATE   CALS BURNED

MEASUREMENTS

NECK	
R BICEP	
L BICEP	
CHEST	
WAIST	
HIPS	
R THIGH	
L THIGH	
CALF	

NOTES/NUTUITION

DATE: _____   S M T W T F S   WEIGHT: _____

MUSCLE GROUP: _____ START TIME: _____ FINISH TIME: _____

STRENGTH TRAINING   HOW I FEEL: 😀 😊 😐 😟 😣   WATER: 8oz. 8oz. 8oz. 8oz. 8oz. 8oz. 8oz. 8oz. 8oz. 8oz.

- [ ] UPPER BODY
- [ ] LOWER BODY
- [ ] ABS

EXERCISE	SET	1	2	3	4	5	6
	REPS						
	WEIGHT						
	REPS						
	WEIGHT						
	REPS						
	WEIGHT						
	REPS						
	WEIGHT						
	REPS						
	WEIGHT						
	REPS						
	WEIGHT						
	REPS						
	WEIGHT						
	REPS						
	WEIGHT						
	REPS						
	WEIGHT						
	REPS						
	WEIGHT						

CARDIO	TIME	DISTANCE	HEART RATE	CALS BURNED

NOTES/NUTUITION

MEASUREMENTS

NECK	
R BICEP	
L BICEP	
CHEST	
WAIST	
HIPS	
R THIGH	
L THIGH	
CALF	

DATE: _____ S M T W T F S   WEIGHT: _____

MUSCLE GROUP: _____ START TIME: _____ FINISH TIME: _____

STRENGTH TRAINING   HOW I FEEL: 😊 😌 😐 😣 😫   WATER: 8oz 8oz 8oz 8oz 8oz 8oz 8oz 8oz

☐ UPPER BODY   ☐ LOWER BODY   ☐ ABS

EXERCISE	SET	1	2	3	4	5	6
	REPS						
	WEIGHT						
	REPS						
	WEIGHT						
	REPS						
	WEIGHT						
	REPS						
	WEIGHT						
	REPS						
	WEIGHT						
	REPS						
	WEIGHT						
	REPS						
	WEIGHT						
	REPS						
	WEIGHT						
	REPS						
	WEIGHT						
	REPS						
	WEIGHT						

CARDIO	TIME	DISTANCE	HEART RATE	CALS BURNED

MEASUREMENTS

NECK	
R BICEP	
L BICEP	
CHEST	
WAIST	
HIPS	
R THIGH	
L THIGH	
CALF	

NOTES/NUTUITION

DATE: _____ S M T W T F S   WEIGHT: _____

MUSCLE GROUP: _____ START TIME: _____ FINISH TIME: _____

STRENGTH TRAINING   HOW I FEEL: 😊 😄 😐 😖 😣   WATER: 8oz. 8oz. 8oz. 8oz. 8oz. 8oz. 8oz. 8oz.

☐ UPPER BODY   ☐ LOWER BODY   ☐ ABS

EXERCISE	SET	1	2	3	4	5	6
	REPS						
	WEIGHT						
	REPS						
	WEIGHT						
	REPS						
	WEIGHT						
	REPS						
	WEIGHT						
	REPS						
	WEIGHT						
	REPS						
	WEIGHT						
	REPS						
	WEIGHT						
	REPS						
	WEIGHT						
	REPS						
	WEIGHT						
	REPS						
	WEIGHT						

CARDIO	TIME	DISTANCE	HEART RATE	CALS BURNED

MEASUREMENTS

NECK	
R BICEP	
L BICEP	
CHEST	
WAIST	
HIPS	
R THIGH	
L THIGH	
CALF	

NOTES/NUTUITION

DATE: _____ ☐ ☐ ☐ ☐ ☐ ☐ ☐   WEIGHT: _____
             S M T W T F S

MUSCLE GROUP: _____ START TIME: _____ FINISH TIME: _____

STRENGTH TRAINING   HOW I FEEL: 😊 😌 😐 😒 😣   WATER: 8oz. 8oz. 8oz. 8oz. 8oz. 8oz. 8oz. 8oz.

☐ UPPER BODY   ☐ LOWER BODY   ☐ ABS

EXERCISE	SET	1	2	3	4	5	6
	REPS						
	WEIGHT						
	REPS						
	WEIGHT						
	REPS						
	WEIGHT						
	REPS						
	WEIGHT						
	REPS						
	WEIGHT						
	REPS						
	WEIGHT						
	REPS						
	WEIGHT						
	REPS						
	WEIGHT						
	REPS						
	WEIGHT						
	REPS						
	WEIGHT						

CARDIO	TIME	DISTANCE	HEART RATE	CALS BURNED

MEASUREMENTS

NECK	
R BICEP	
L BICEP	
CHEST	
WAIST	
HIPS	
R THIGH	
L THIGH	
CALF	

NOTES/NUTUITION

DATE: _____ ☐ ☐ ☐ ☐ ☐ ☐ ☐ WEIGHT: _____
S M T W T F S

MUSCLE GROUP: _____ START TIME: _____ FINISH TIME: _____

STRENGTH TRAINING   HOW I FEEL: 😀 😊 😐 😟 😣   WATER: 8oz 8oz 8oz 8oz 8oz 8oz 8oz 8oz

☐ UPPER BODY   ☐ LOWER BODY   ☐ ABS

EXERCISE	SET	1	2	3	4	5	6
	REPS						
	WEIGHT						
	REPS						
	WEIGHT						
	REPS						
	WEIGHT						
	REPS						
	WEIGHT						
	REPS						
	WEIGHT						
	REPS						
	WEIGHT						
	REPS						
	WEIGHT						
	REPS						
	WEIGHT						
	REPS						
	WEIGHT						
	REPS						
	WEIGHT						

CARDIO	TIME	DISTANCE	HEART RATE	CALS BURNED

MEASUREMENTS

NECK	
R BICEP	
L BICEP	
CHEST	
WAIST	
HIPS	
R THIGH	
L THIGH	
CALF	

NOTES/NUTUITION

DATE: _____   S M T W T F S   WEIGHT: _____

MUSCLE GROUP: _____   START TIME: _____   FINISH TIME: _____

STRENGTH TRAINING   HOW I FEEL: 😊 😉 😐 😟 😣   WATER: 8oz 8oz 8oz 8oz 8oz 8oz 8oz 8oz

- [ ] UPPER BODY
- [ ] LOWER BODY
- [ ] ABS

EXERCISE	SET	1	2	3	4	5	6
	REPS						
	WEIGHT						
	REPS						
	WEIGHT						
	REPS						
	WEIGHT						
	REPS						
	WEIGHT						
	REPS						
	WEIGHT						
	REPS						
	WEIGHT						
	REPS						
	WEIGHT						
	REPS						
	WEIGHT						
	REPS						
	WEIGHT						
	REPS						
	WEIGHT						

CARDIO	TIME	DISTANCE	HEART RATE	CALS BURNED

NOTES/NUTUITION

MEASUREMENTS	
NECK	
R BICEP	
L BICEP	
CHEST	
WAIST	
HIPS	
R THIGH	
L THIGH	
CALF	

DATE: _____   S M T W T F S   WEIGHT: _____

MUSCLE GROUP: _____   START TIME: _____   FINISH TIME: _____

STRENGTH TRAINING   HOW I FEEL: 😊 😌 😐 😕 😣   WATER: 8oz 8oz 8oz 8oz 8oz 8oz 8oz 8oz 8oz

- [ ] UPPER BODY
- [ ] LOWER BODY
- [ ] ABS

EXERCISE	SET	1	2	3	4	5	6
	REPS						
	WEIGHT						
	REPS						
	WEIGHT						
	REPS						
	WEIGHT						
	REPS						
	WEIGHT						
	REPS						
	WEIGHT						
	REPS						
	WEIGHT						
	REPS						
	WEIGHT						
	REPS						
	WEIGHT						
	REPS						
	WEIGHT						
	REPS						
	WEIGHT						

CARDIO	TIME	DISTANCE	HEART RATE	CALS BURNED

MEASUREMENTS

NECK	
R BICEP	
L BICEP	
CHEST	
WAIST	
HIPS	
R THIGH	
L THIGH	
CALF	

NOTES/NUTUITION

DATE: _____ S M T W T F S   WEIGHT: _____

MUSCLE GROUP: _____ START TIME: _____ FINISH TIME: _____

STRENGTH TRAINING   HOW I FEEL: 😀 😊 😐 😫 😖   WATER: 8 oz. 8 oz. 8 oz. 8 oz. 8 oz. 8 oz. 8 oz. 8 oz. 8 oz.

- [ ] UPPER BODY
- [ ] LOWER BODY
- [ ] ABS

EXERCISE	SET	1	2	3	4	5	6
	REPS						
	WEIGHT						
	REPS						
	WEIGHT						
	REPS						
	WEIGHT						
	REPS						
	WEIGHT						
	REPS						
	WEIGHT						
	REPS						
	WEIGHT						
	REPS						
	WEIGHT						
	REPS						
	WEIGHT						
	REPS						
	WEIGHT						
	REPS						
	WEIGHT						

CARDIO	TIME	DISTANCE	HEART RATE	CALS BURNED

MEASUREMENTS

NECK	
R BICEP	
L BICEP	
CHEST	
WAIST	
HIPS	
R THIGH	
L THIGH	
CALF	

NOTES/NUTUITION

DATE: _____ S M T W T F S   WEIGHT: _____

MUSCLE GROUP: _____ START TIME: _____ FINISH TIME: _____

STRENGTH TRAINING   HOW I FEEL: 😊 😌 😐 😕 😠   WATER: 8oz 8oz 8oz 8oz 8oz 8oz 8oz 8oz

☐ UPPER BODY   ☐ LOWER BODY   ☐ ABS

EXERCISE	SET	1	2	3	4	5	6
	REPS						
	WEIGHT						
	REPS						
	WEIGHT						
	REPS						
	WEIGHT						
	REPS						
	WEIGHT						
	REPS						
	WEIGHT						
	REPS						
	WEIGHT						
	REPS						
	WEIGHT						
	REPS						
	WEIGHT						
	REPS						
	WEIGHT						
	REPS						
	WEIGHT						

CARDIO	TIME	DISTANCE	HEART RATE	CALS BURNED

NOTES/NUTUITION

MEASUREMENTS

NECK	
R BICEP	
L BICEP	
CHEST	
WAIST	
HIPS	
R THIGH	
L THIGH	
CALF	

DATE: _____ ☐ ☐ ☐ ☐ ☐ ☐ ☐ WEIGHT: _____
                                S M T W T F S

MUSCLE GROUP: _____ START TIME: _____ FINISH TIME: _____

STRENGTH TRAINING   HOW I FEEL: 😀 🙂 😐 😕 😣   WATER: 8oz. 8oz. 8oz. 8oz. 8oz. 8oz. 8oz. 8oz.

☐ UPPER BODY   ☐ LOWER BODY   ☐ ABS

EXERCISE	SET	1	2	3	4	5	6
	REPS						
	WEIGHT						
	REPS						
	WEIGHT						
	REPS						
	WEIGHT						
	REPS						
	WEIGHT						
	REPS						
	WEIGHT						
	REPS						
	WEIGHT						
	REPS						
	WEIGHT						
	REPS						
	WEIGHT						
	REPS						
	WEIGHT						
	REPS						
	WEIGHT						

CARDIO	TIME	DISTANCE	HEART RATE	CALS BURNED

MEASUREMENTS

NECK	
R BICEP	
L BICEP	
CHEST	
WAIST	
HIPS	
R THIGH	
L THIGH	
CALF	

NOTES/NUTUITION

DATE: _____ S M T W T F S   WEIGHT: _____

MUSCLE GROUP: _____ START TIME: _____ FINISH TIME: _____

STRENGTH TRAINING HOW I FEEL: 😀 😊 😐 😣 😠   WATER: 8oz. 8oz. 8oz. 8oz. 8oz. 8oz. 8oz. 8oz.

- [ ] UPPER BODY
- [ ] LOWER BODY
- [ ] ABS

EXERCISE	SET	1	2	3	4	5	6
	REPS						
	WEIGHT						
	REPS						
	WEIGHT						
	REPS						
	WEIGHT						
	REPS						
	WEIGHT						
	REPS						
	WEIGHT						
	REPS						
	WEIGHT						
	REPS						
	WEIGHT						
	REPS						
	WEIGHT						
	REPS						
	WEIGHT						
	REPS						
	WEIGHT						

CARDIO	TIME	DISTANCE	HEART RATE	CALS BURNED

MEASUREMENTS

NECK	
R BICEP	
L BICEP	
CHEST	
WAIST	
HIPS	
R THIGH	
L THIGH	
CALF	

NOTES/NUTUITION

DATE: _____ ☐ ☐ ☐ ☐ ☐ ☐ ☐ WEIGHT: _____
　　　　　　　　　　　 S M T W T F S

MUSCLE GROUP: _____ START TIME: _____ FINISH TIME: _____

STRENGTH TRAINING　　HOW I FEEL: 😃 😊 😐 😟 😣　　WATER: 8oz. 8oz. 8oz. 8oz. 8oz. 8oz. 8oz. 8oz.

☐ UPPER BODY　　　　☐ LOWER BODY　　　　☐ ABS

EXERCISE	SET	1	2	3	4	5	6
	REPS						
	WEIGHT						
	REPS						
	WEIGHT						
	REPS						
	WEIGHT						
	REPS						
	WEIGHT						
	REPS						
	WEIGHT						
	REPS						
	WEIGHT						
	REPS						
	WEIGHT						
	REPS						
	WEIGHT						
	REPS						
	WEIGHT						
	REPS						
	WEIGHT						

CARDIO	TIME	DISTANCE	HEART RATE	CALS BURNED

MEASUREMENTS

NECK	
R BICEP	
L BICEP	
CHEST	
WAIST	
HIPS	
R THIGH	
L THIGH	
CALF	

NOTES/NUTUITION

DATE: _____ S M T W T F S   WEIGHT: _____

MUSCLE GROUP: _____ START TIME: _____ FINISH TIME: _____

STRENGTH TRAINING   HOW I FEEL: 😃 🙂 😐 😟 😣   WATER: 8oz 8oz 8oz 8oz 8oz 8oz 8oz 8oz 8oz 8oz

☐ UPPER BODY   ☐ LOWER BODY   ☐ ABS

EXERCISE	SET	1	2	3	4	5	6
	REPS						
	WEIGHT						
	REPS						
	WEIGHT						
	REPS						
	WEIGHT						
	REPS						
	WEIGHT						
	REPS						
	WEIGHT						
	REPS						
	WEIGHT						
	REPS						
	WEIGHT						
	REPS						
	WEIGHT						
	REPS						
	WEIGHT						
	REPS						
	WEIGHT						

CARDIO	TIME	DISTANCE	HEART RATE	CALS BURNED

MEASUREMENTS

NECK	
R BICEP	
L BICEP	
CHEST	
WAIST	
HIPS	
R THIGH	
L THIGH	
CALF	

NOTES/NUTUITION

DATE: _____ ☐S ☐M ☐T ☐W ☐T ☐F ☐S   WEIGHT: _____

MUSCLE GROUP: _____ START TIME: _____ FINISH TIME: _____

STRENGTH TRAINING   HOW I FEEL: 😀 😊 😐 😟 😣   WATER: 8oz. 8oz. 8oz. 8oz. 8oz. 8oz. 8oz. 8oz.

☐ UPPER BODY   ☐ LOWER BODY   ☐ ABS

EXERCISE	SET	1	2	3	4	5	6
	REPS						
	WEIGHT						
	REPS						
	WEIGHT						
	REPS						
	WEIGHT						
	REPS						
	WEIGHT						
	REPS						
	WEIGHT						
	REPS						
	WEIGHT						
	REPS						
	WEIGHT						
	REPS						
	WEIGHT						
	REPS						
	WEIGHT						
	REPS						
	WEIGHT						

CARDIO	TIME	DISTANCE	HEART RATE	CALS BURNED

NOTES/NUTUITION

MEASUREMENTS

NECK	
R BICEP	
L BICEP	
CHEST	
WAIST	
HIPS	
R THIGH	
L THIGH	
CALF	

DATE: _____ S M T W T F S WEIGHT: _____

MUSCLE GROUP: _____ START TIME: _____ FINISH TIME: _____

STRENGTH TRAINING HOW I FEEL: 😊 😌 😐 😕 😠 WATER: 8oz. 8oz. 8oz. 8oz. 8oz. 8oz. 8oz. 8oz. 8oz. 8oz.

☐ UPPER BODY   ☐ LOWER BODY   ☐ ABS

EXERCISE	SET	1	2	3	4	5	6
	REPS						
	WEIGHT						
	REPS						
	WEIGHT						
	REPS						
	WEIGHT						
	REPS						
	WEIGHT						
	REPS						
	WEIGHT						
	REPS						
	WEIGHT						
	REPS						
	WEIGHT						
	REPS						
	WEIGHT						
	REPS						
	WEIGHT						
	REPS						
	WEIGHT						

CARDIO	TIME	DISTANCE	HEART RATE	CALS BURNED

MEASUREMENTS

NECK	
R BICEP	
L BICEP	
CHEST	
WAIST	
HIPS	
R THIGH	
L THIGH	
CALF	

NOTES/NUTUITION

DATE: _____ S M T W T F S   WEIGHT: _____

MUSCLE GROUP: _____ START TIME: _____ FINISH TIME: _____

STRENGTH TRAINING   HOW I FEEL: 😊 😌 😐 😣 😫   WATER: 8oz. 8oz. 8oz. 8oz. 8oz. 8oz. 8oz. 8oz.

- [ ] UPPER BODY
- [ ] LOWER BODY
- [ ] ABS

EXERCISE	SET	1	2	3	4	5	6
	REPS						
	WEIGHT						
	REPS						
	WEIGHT						
	REPS						
	WEIGHT						
	REPS						
	WEIGHT						
	REPS						
	WEIGHT						
	REPS						
	WEIGHT						
	REPS						
	WEIGHT						
	REPS						
	WEIGHT						
	REPS						
	WEIGHT						
	REPS						
	WEIGHT						

CARDIO	TIME	DISTANCE	HEART RATE	CALS BURNED

MEASUREMENTS

NECK	
R BICEP	
L BICEP	
CHEST	
WAIST	
HIPS	
R THIGH	
L THIGH	
CALF	

NOTES/NUTUITION

DATE: _____ ☐ ☐ ☐ ☐ ☐ ☐ ☐ WEIGHT: _____
             S M T W T F S

MUSCLE GROUP: _____ START TIME: _____ FINISH TIME: _____

STRENGTH TRAINING   HOW I FEEL: 😊 😄 😐 😣 😖   WATER: 8oz 8oz 8oz 8oz 8oz 8oz 8oz 8oz

☐ UPPER BODY   ☐ LOWER BODY   ☐ ABS

EXERCISE	SET	1	2	3	4	5	6
	REPS						
	WEIGHT						
	REPS						
	WEIGHT						
	REPS						
	WEIGHT						
	REPS						
	WEIGHT						
	REPS						
	WEIGHT						
	REPS						
	WEIGHT						
	REPS						
	WEIGHT						
	REPS						
	WEIGHT						
	REPS						
	WEIGHT						
	REPS						
	WEIGHT						

CARDIO	TIME	DISTANCE	HEART RATE	CALS BURNED

MEASUREMENTS

NECK	
R BICEP	
L BICEP	
CHEST	
WAIST	
HIPS	
R THIGH	
L THIGH	
CALF	

NOTES/NUTUITION

DATE: _____ ☐S ☐M ☐T ☐W ☐T ☐F ☐S   WEIGHT: _____

MUSCLE GROUP: _____ START TIME: _____ FINISH TIME: _____

STRENGTH TRAINING   HOW I FEEL: 😊 😌 😐 😣 😫   WATER: 8oz 8oz 8oz 8oz 8oz 8oz 8oz 8oz

☐ UPPER BODY   ☐ LOWER BODY   ☐ ABS

EXERCISE	SET	1	2	3	4	5	6
	REPS						
	WEIGHT						
	REPS						
	WEIGHT						
	REPS						
	WEIGHT						
	REPS						
	WEIGHT						
	REPS						
	WEIGHT						
	REPS						
	WEIGHT						
	REPS						
	WEIGHT						
	REPS						
	WEIGHT						
	REPS						
	WEIGHT						
	REPS						
	WEIGHT						

CARDIO	TIME	DISTANCE	HEART RATE	CALS BURNED

NOTES/NUTUITION

MEASUREMENTS	
NECK	
R BICEP	
L BICEP	
CHEST	
WAIST	
HIPS	
R THIGH	
L THIGH	
CALF	

DATE: _____ ☐ ☐ ☐ ☐ ☐ ☐ ☐ WEIGHT: _____
                                 S M T W T F S

MUSCLE GROUP: _____ START TIME: _____ FINISH TIME: _____

STRENGTH TRAINING   HOW I FEEL: 😊 😌 😐 😟 😣   WATER: 8oz 8oz 8oz 8oz 8oz 8oz 8oz 8oz

☐ UPPER BODY   ☐ LOWER BODY   ☐ ABS

EXERCISE	SET	1	2	3	4	5	6
	REPS						
	WEIGHT						
	REPS						
	WEIGHT						
	REPS						
	WEIGHT						
	REPS						
	WEIGHT						
	REPS						
	WEIGHT						
	REPS						
	WEIGHT						
	REPS						
	WEIGHT						
	REPS						
	WEIGHT						
	REPS						
	WEIGHT						
	REPS						
	WEIGHT						

CARDIO	TIME	DISTANCE	HEART RATE	CALS BURNED

MEASUREMENTS

NECK	
R BICEP	
L BICEP	
CHEST	
WAIST	
HIPS	
R THIGH	
L THIGH	
CALF	

NOTES/NUTUITION

DATE: _____ ☐ ☐ ☐ ☐ ☐ ☐ ☐   WEIGHT: _____
                                                   S M T W T F S

MUSCLE GROUP: _____ START TIME: _____ FINISH TIME: _____

STRENGTH TRAINING   HOW I FEEL: 😀 😊 😐 😒 😣   WATER: 8oz. 8oz. 8oz. 8oz. 8oz. 8oz. 8oz. 8oz.

☐ UPPER BODY   ☐ LOWER BODY   ☐ ABS

EXERCISE	SET	1	2	3	4	5	6
	REPS						
	WEIGHT						
	REPS						
	WEIGHT						
	REPS						
	WEIGHT						
	REPS						
	WEIGHT						
	REPS						
	WEIGHT						
	REPS						
	WEIGHT						
	REPS						
	WEIGHT						
	REPS						
	WEIGHT						
	REPS						
	WEIGHT						
	REPS						
	WEIGHT						

CARDIO	TIME	DISTANCE	HEART RATE	CALS BURNED

MEASUREMENTS

NECK	
R BICEP	
L BICEP	
CHEST	
WAIST	
HIPS	
R THIGH	
L THIGH	
CALF	

NOTES/NUTUITION

Made in the USA
Coppell, TX
11 December 2021